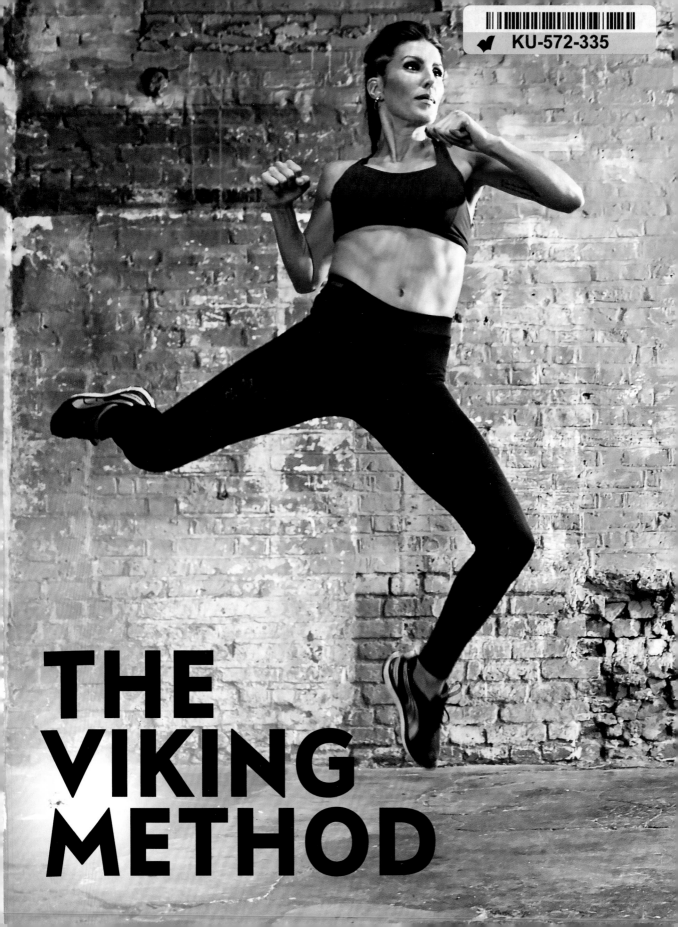

THE VIKING METHOD

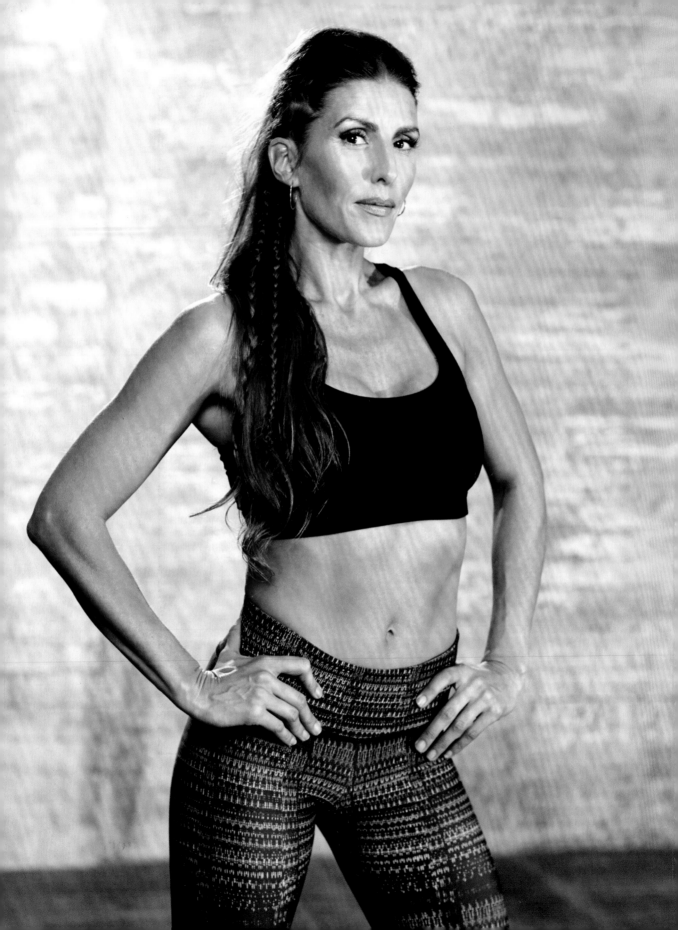

Items should be returned on or before the last date shown below. Items not already requested by other borrowers may be renewed in person, in writing or by telephone. To renew, please quote the number on the barcode label. To renew online a PIN is required. This can be requested at your local library.
Renew online @ **www.dublincitypubliclibraries.ie**
Fines charged for overdue items will include postage incurred in recovery. Damage to or loss of items will be charged to the borrower.

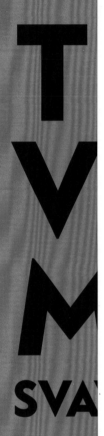

Date Due	Date Due	Date Due

LIFE

FOR MY PAST, WHICH MADE ME DREAM AND DARE AND NEVER SURRENDER. AND FOR MY FUTURE, WHICH INSPIRES ME, PUSHES ME AND STRIVES ME TO CONSTANTLY BECOME MORE.

THIS BOOK IS FOR MY MOTHER AND FOR MY DAUGHTER.

PENGUIN LIFE

UK | USA | Canada | Ireland | Australia
India | New Zealand | South Africa

Penguin Life is part of the Penguin Random House group of companies
whose addresses can be found at global.penguinrandomhouse.com.

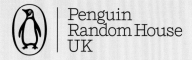

Penguin
Random House
UK

First published 2019
001

Copyright © Svava Sigbertsdottir 2019

The moral right of the author has been asserted

Printed and bound in China by C&C Offset Printing Co., Ltd

A CIP catalogue record for this book is available from the British Library

ISBN: 978–0–241–30949–0
Design and art direction: Smith & Gilmour
Photographer (portraits): Philip North-Coombes
Photographer (exercise): Sam Riley
Photographer (food): Smith & Gilmour Ltd
Food stylist: Vicki Keppel-Compton

www.greenpenguin.co.uk

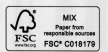

MIX
Paper from
responsible sources
FSC® C018179

Penguin Random House is committed to a
sustainable future for our business, our readers
and our planet. This book is made from Forest
Stewardship Council® certified paper.

CONTENTS

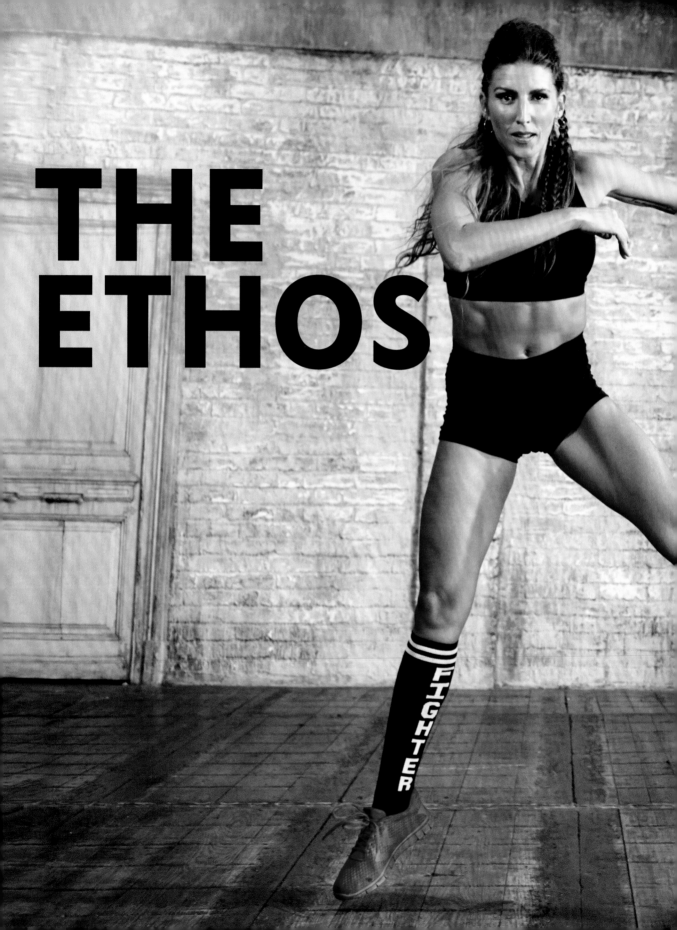

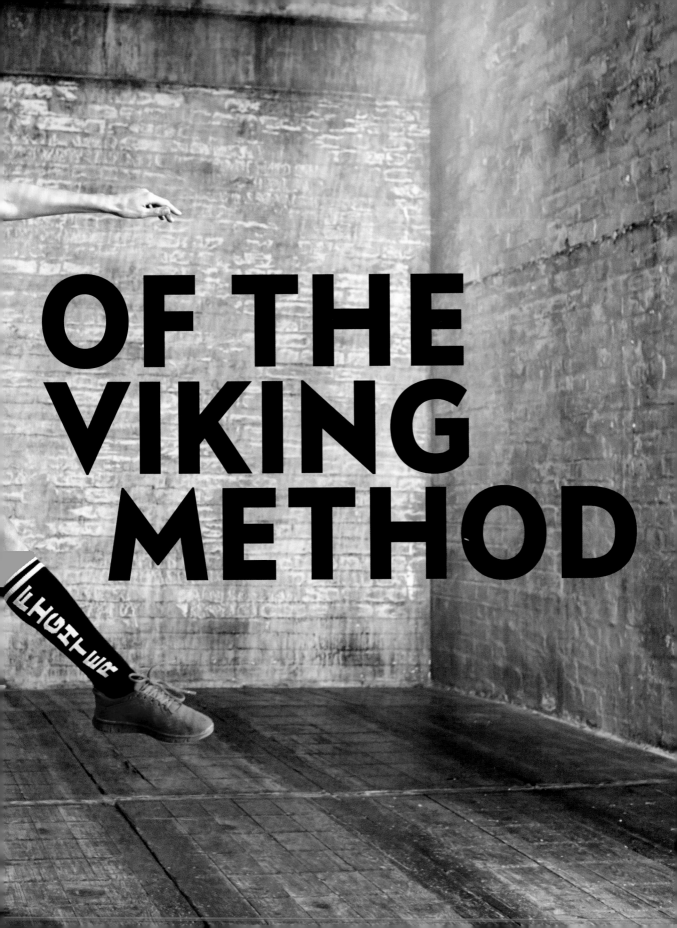

OF THE
VIKING
METHOD

VIKING MANTRA #1

I LIVE IN AN AGE OF APPROVAL.
BUT I STAND APART FROM IT.
I LIKE MYSELF.
WHY DO I NEED LIKES?
I SEE MYSELF. WHY DO I NEED A MIRROR?
I AM MY OWN SOURCE OF POWER.
THERE'S NO CHANGE I CANNOT FACE,
NO CHALLENGE I CANNOT MEET,
NO TERRITORY I CANNOT CONQUER.
THE GOODNESS I WANT FROM
THE WORLD, I TAKE.
I WRITE MY OWN VALUES.
I STEER MY OWN SHIP.
I AM A VIKING.

THE INSIDE OUT APPROACH OF THE VIKING METHOD

'JUST GO TO THE GYM AND EAT HEALTHILY. THAT'S IT.'

How often have you heard that this is the simple secret to health and happiness – like it's that easy? And if you don't work out regularly and eat your greens, obviously this is because you are lazy, weak and just not trying hard enough.

But if staying in great health is so easy, why is it that so many of us struggle? What is stopping people from achieving their optimum health and happiness? The problem is that most fitness methods, trainers and the media fail to mention the most important part of a healthy lifestyle: your mentality. They approach fitness from the viewpoint of what it looks like externally. And that doesn't work in the long run. Your internal state is at the root of everything. Your actions and your lack of actions, your good and your bad choices and your level of self-worth all stem from your inner state. Therefore, you need to make that strong and healthy, to support and maintain any positive change you seek.

The Viking Method is different because it incorporates all of you: your mental and your physical strength. Furthermore, it starts from the inside, and works its way out.

The Viking Method is three-fold: Your mentality. Your training. Your nutrition.

The Viking Method is not about just getting you ready for the beach or crash-dieting in January to get your weight down after Christmas excess. Those are not our goals. They are too small, too fleeting. We have much bigger, deeper and more long-lasting goals.

The mental coaching, exercise programme and nutritional advice in these pages are all the tools you need in order to make change happen. I am not just giving you two or three tools – I am giving you the whole toolbox.

THINK
LIKE A VIKING

» Vikings are fully in control of their mind, of their body and of their life.

» Vikings do not allow situations, other people, or even themselves, to hold them back. They know what they want and they know that only they have the power to make it happen.

» Vikings do not say 'I should,' they say, 'I will.'

» Following this method will make you stronger, more powerful, faster, more agile, more energetic, confident and more content. The by-product of the Viking Method is a great-looking body, which you will get, but that is not the focus. The focus is on you, and what you do.

» What you put in is what you get out, and Vikings know that their results will be great – not just in their training but in all they do in life.

TRAIN
LIKE A VIKING

» Vikings train using their own body weight along with free weights.

» Vikings always train to their maximum. They give it their all. Not to prove someone else wrong, but to prove themselves right.

» Vikings train five times a week for just 30 minutes, though during that time they push themselves to their limit and beyond.

» Exercises are grouped together in a specific way: functional dynamic movements with functional static movements, carried out within a certain time frame/repetition. This promotes greater lean tissue building and further use of energy and oxygen, increasing fat utilization and heightening your metabolic rate (the rate at which your body burns energy).

» The Method will make you mentally more resilient and confident as you progress through the training programme and perform exercises you never thought you could do.

» The result: a strong, toned body with long, lean muscles, great balance and correct posture – and a powerful mind.

EAT
LIKE A VIKING

» Vikings eat a clean, simple, Nordic diet.

» Vikings value the quality and nutritional value of what they eat rather than the presentation or colour coordination.

» Vikings eat food that fuels and powers their strong body and mind.

» The Viking Method diet is no frills, with no difficult recipes, no travelling long distances for special ingredients. It's healthy, realistic and delicious.

» The recipes in this book include poultry, fish, meat, vegetables, fruit, berries, nuts, seeds, oats and other complex carbs.

» What is key to the Viking Method diet is that your nutrition will differ on training days and rest days. On training days, you should have a higher carbohydrate intake to fuel your training and recovery: as you are doing high-intensity training, your body will utilize your carbs for energy and to replenish your muscles instead of converting them into fat.

» Carbohydrates are split into two categories: Always Carbs (non-starchy veggies and fibrous fruits) and Sometimes Carbs (brown rice, oats, potatoes, lentils and beans). As these names suggest, Always Carbs can be eaten every day and Sometimes Carbs are for training days. Training days start with complex Sometimes Carbs for breakfast, and you also have Sometimes Carbs in your Post-training Meal, to replenish energy after you've exercised.

VIKING MANTRA #2

GREATNESS IS NOT SOMETHING THAT IS LIMITED OR UNOBTAINABLE OR RESERVED. GREATNESS IS NOT SOMETHING THAT YOU ARE EITHER BORN WITH OR YOU ARE NOT. GREATNESS IS NOT SOMETHING THAT YOU CAN RECEIVE AUTOMATICALLY THROUGH CLASS, RACE, RELIGION OR MONEY. GREATNESS IS CREATED. IT'S BUILT. IT'S SHARPENED. IT'S FORGED. IT'S NURTURED. BY YOU. FROM WITHIN YOU. GREATNESS IS THERE FOR YOUR TAKING. TAKE IT. TODAY. GREATNESS IS YOURS.

SVAVA'S SAGA

Once, when I was little, I came home from school and told my mum that someone had said I was stupid.

My mum said: 'If someone says you are a car, are you a car?'

'No,' I said. 'Of course I'm not.'

To which my mum replied, 'Exactly.'

I come from Iceland, the oldest of three siblings. We were always allowed to be who we wanted to be, dress how we wanted to, and were encouraged to give everything a try. My brother wanted to be Superman, so he went everywhere with his underwear over his trousers and a tea towel around his neck. My sister dressed like a fairy princess, never leaving the house without at least ten rings and necklaces. I played handball and football for my hometown sports club and the only thing I wore was my team's tracksuit, and only that tracksuit, for years. Apart from at Christmas.

I have always trained hard. I love sports. I love practising and bettering a skill. I love the competitiveness, the power, and most of all the mental strength. People in Iceland are huge on sports. Love of sports is ingrained in you as a child and that carries through into your adulthood. Whether it was snowing or sunny, during PE, we ran outside. No one cared if it was minus degrees and you had wet hair after swimming lessons. The attitude was: bring a hat and get on with it, and this makes you tough. It makes you feel like you can do anything and overcome anything. The World's Strongest Man was always a massive thing in Iceland. When I was growing up, having a strong, capable, Viking body was something to aspire to. If you could drag a car around and lift some massive stones, you were the coolest kid in school.

I was encouraged by my parents to be the best that I could be in all the things I did. If I didn't do well, I was told that I didn't. Nothing was sugar-coated. Equally, when I did well, I was praised. But my mother did it in such a way that it was always just my actions that were being assessed. I never felt judged or not good enough, or that I needed to perform in a certain way to be valued. What my mother did was teach me that I steer the ship when it comes to my self-worth. I set my own bar.

'I dare, I can, I will.' This was what my mum said with me before every game, every show, anything that required bravery and ability.

My parents praised me for being smart, strong, powerful, kind, funny and hard-working. These are the things I was taught to value. I was never praised for my appearance. How my body looked was not made into a big deal and therefore I never felt that I equalled my body. If I gained or lost weight unhealthily, my parents would speak to me about it in a matter-of-fact way so that it never impacted negatively on my self-esteem.

When I was seventeen, I got pregnant with my daughter, Raven. Her father and I were so happy about it. For a while we lived together in Iceland in a flat near my parents' house, but in 2004 I split up with Raven's dad and decided to move to London to go to a performing arts school. At first Raven, who was six at the time, couldn't come with me and stayed with her dad for a while. It was extremely difficult and to this day I still carry the guilt with me, but I did it to make a better life for us, and knowing this gave me the drive and determination that I continue to carry with me today.

While I was studying, we used to dance for hours every day. Ballet, contemporary, tap – but nothing gave me that tight, lean, athletic body nor the power, strength and agility that I wanted. So I started to develop my own method, drawing on my roots from Iceland – the love for training no matter where and in all weathers, along with the mental toughness required – and combined it with my training – my core and balance work, kickboxing, dancing and my mental practices – and created the Viking Method, using myself as my first client. I completely changed inside and out: on the outside, I became lean and toned, with long muscles full of power and strength. And on the inside I became more resilient, bolder and full of belief in myself and my abilities.

During the time when I created and set up the Viking Method, I had nothing. It was a tough time personally and financially, and living in a country without all my family and closest friends I felt quite alone in the world. Of course, I had Raven with me by then, which gave me the greatest love, but I am her mother, and I take care of her, not the other way around. During this time, I developed the three elements of the Viking Method, as what I was doing – my own training, nutrition and later my mental training – saved me. Everything stood and fell with me; there was no one to fall back on, complain to or help ease the load. The Method made me truly realize my own strength, as my situation didn't get the best of me – instead, it actually made me better. It helped me to understand that I was completely in control of my life and that what I do will result in what I get.

I decided to fully utilize this realization, by doing what I needed to make the vision I had for my Method and for myself a reality. I came up

against many obstacles and setbacks while getting the Method up and running. The constant 'nos' were draining. But not defeating. They actually kept me going, because I was not going to stop before that 'yes' would roll in. If you get through the 'nos', if you keep on going and don't take 'no' as your answer, you will eventually get a 'yes'. My Viking training kept me going and kept me focused. It gave me a physical outlet, encouraged mental clarity and constantly reminded me that there is nothing that I cannot do. As my body became stronger, and constantly surprised me with its progress and what I could achieve, my resolve to be successful in my business became just as strong.

That 'yes' came when Nicole Scherzinger came to London to be a judge on The X Factor and I thought that she might not bring her trainer from the US with her. So I emailed her, she replied and I ended up training Nicole a few days later. She loved the Method and I trained her throughout The X Factor and continue to do so whenever she is in London.

My goal was to create a Method that would help people realize how badass they are. Life is about feeling good and being happy in your own skin, and I cannot explain how much joy it gives me that I play a part in helping people to feel like that. I am so proud of every single person who is doing the Viking Method programme. You are all amazing. It takes guts to make a change, to decide that you deserve much more. It takes guts to stand up and actually go for it. So, welcome to the greatest clan, my dearest Viking. I am so happy that you are here!

THE 12 CODES OF THE VIKING METHOD

#1
YOU ARE NOT YOUR BODY.

Stop letting your body dictate you – how you feel about yourself, the value you give to yourself, the love you have for yourself. You are so much more than you give yourself credit for.

Just like fashion changes, so does body fashion. Now big behinds are said to be the ultimate component for self-contentment, and if you don't have one, you are not deemed attractive. This was not the case some years ago, when neat, small bottoms were in vogue. The way you view your body cannot be dictated by the way the outside world views bodies. Your body is such an amazing tool. Be grateful to it, train it and take wonderful care of it, but at the same time, never mistake it for you.

#2
GET COMFORTABLE WITH BEING UNCOMFORTABLE.

Change happens in the uncomfortable zone: where you feel like you cannot give any more but still power through. Where your mind is saying 'no more' but still you do not quit.

When doing an exercise, if the last three reps (repetitions) are not a great struggle, you need to make it harder. Use heavier weights, go faster, go deeper or engage your muscles more. Be on the verge of failing and push through. Or fail. Then one day you won't fail, because you made a change happen by training to your max.

#3
QUALITY OVER QUANTITY.

Make every exercise count. In the Viking Method, there are no time fillers, like jumping jacks. It is so important that you know how to do each exercise and why you are doing it, what muscles you are using, how your posture should be during the exercise, your starting point and your end point. You should never just do the movement, but should always consciously engage your muscles.

When you are in a plank (see page 57) and reach one arm forward, don't just reach one arm forward. Get your shoulders back, engage your core (see page 18), control the arm as you extend it forward, as well as watching that your hipbone is facing the floor, keeping that contraction in your core. Be connected to your body the whole time you are training. You recruit more muscle fibres by thinking about what you're doing and being actively present instead of just doing the movement. When you train consciously, you get more out of fewer reps.

Don't confuse longevity with a job well done. The length of your workout doesn't matter; whether you do the exercise properly does.

#4
YOU ARE YOUR OWN KEEPER.

The sooner you realize that you are in control, the sooner your life will change for the better. It can be a little scary to realize that it all comes down to you, but with that realization also comes great power.

You cannot change anything you have no control over, but you do have control over yourself and your life. Making excuses, blaming others, allotting power to other people, will only make you less and bring less to your life. Take your power back. It has always been yours, you just forgot that.

Start small. You don't have to begin by walking out of your job that gives you no joy, which would be overwhelming, to say the least. Instead, start by choosing a small positive change and making it. For example, decide that you will take a healthy lunch with you to work, or that when you look in the mirror in the morning you will say something nice to yourself. Then pat yourself on the back. This will give you confidence in your own power. Then increase the size of your changes.

VIKING MANTRA #3

NOTHING GREAT IS EVER ACHIEVED WITH PARTIAL EFFORT. BUT IF YOU GIVE IT EVERYTHING YOU'VE GOT, THEN THERE IS NOTHING YOU CANNOT ACHIEVE. DON'T LET TIME PASS AND STILL BE IN THE JOB YOU DON'T LIKE, IN THE RELATIONSHIP THAT DOESN'T SATISFY YOU, OR IN A STATE OF BEING, PHYSICALLY AND MENTALLY, THAT YOU ARE NOT CONTENT WITH, JUST BECAUSE IT IS A STRUGGLE TO CHANGE THESE THINGS. IT'S MUCH HARDER TO LIVE A LIFE THAT YOU ARE UNHAPPY WITH. THE STRUGGLE IS WORTH IT. AND SO ARE YOU.

#5
CARBS AFTER YOU TRAIN, ALWAYS.

After you train, your muscles are depleted of energy and need to be replenished. On training days, have slow-releasing carbs for breakfast, such as Overnight Chia Porridge with blueberries and cinnamon (see page 112) or Porridge with sunflower seeds and raspberries (see page 110), and then carbs after you train as well, such as Icelandic Lamb Stew (see page 128) or Pesto Chicken & Sweet Potato One-tray Wonder (see page 124). Ideally, train before one of your main meals so that you can eat straight afterwards.

#6
TRAIN AND EAT FOR YOUR HORMONES.

One of the reasons women tend to have more fat than men is because we have more oestrogen receptors than men have. Oestrogen (the primary female sex hormone that promotes the development and the maintenance of female characteristics in the human body) is crucial for you, but too much or too little oestrogen brings an imbalance that has a huge negative effect. Fat has a very big part in the hormonal system; one of its jobs is to produce oestrogen. Which means that the more fat you have, the more oestrogen you have. Too much oestrogen can slow down your metabolism and cause weight gain; it can block the thyroid and prevent fat being used for energy.

When oestrogen is in balance it works with you; when it's not, it works against you.

Men also have more of the lean tissue-building hormones; therefore it is harder for women to 'tone up'. The more muscles you have, the more energy you use! And that's one of the reasons why resistance training is very important for weight loss.

When Vikings train, it's about tapping into the fat-burning hormones. Not just because they are fat-burning but because they also increase energy levels, build lean tissue, and promote stronger bones plus healthy skin, nails and hair (all those Viking plaits need good hair!). In order for those hormones to be activated, certain things need to happen and certain things need to not happen. Getting the right nutrition is a must, but so is timing your protein, fat and carb intake right, i.e. your macronutrients, to get the most out of them. For the full low-down, go to the Your Hormones chapter (see page 24).

#7
MIND OVER MATTER AND MATTER OVER MIND.

Don't let your mind tell you that you can't. Use your body to prove to yourself that you can. When you train, your mind can play tricks on you. We often tell ourselves that it's too hard, that we are too tired, that we can't finish, or 'Let's just do two sets' instead of the three we planned to do.

Your mind can play tricks on you before you even start training. 'Let's not go today, it's cold outside,' or 'There's laundry and cleaning to do that cannot wait.' I get this, and this is what I do: first of all decide to go training. While you're getting ready, putting on your training gear and packing up your equipment, go over what you will be doing: the programme, repetitions of the exercises, how many sets of each group you will be doing, what you will achieve and so on. Don't allow any emotional thoughts. As you reach the gym or set your equipment out at home, decide that, come hell or high water, you will not finish until you've done what you set out to do. Close your mind off, breathe, count your reps, check your technique and posture, feel your strength and focus on your power. Persevere and never give up. The feeling you get from not stopping just because it gets hard is incredible: that is why we train.

#8
SAY NO TO DAIRY.

Cow's milk is made for calves, not humans. Though milk contains many nutrients, the amounts can vary, and it can also contain high amounts of hormones and growth factors which are not good for humans, among them a growth factor that is strongly linked to the development of many cancers. Cow's milk is high in acid, promotes inflammation, and due to the ratio between calcium and magnesium being too big, it is very difficult for us to absorb the calcium. A Swedish research study published by the *British Medical Journal* in 2014 linked high milk intake with increased mortality and fracture rates and higher levels of oxidative stress. Other research has suggested that cow's dairy can actually weaken the bones due to its acidity (as the bones will release calcium to counteract the acid now in the bloodstream). Avoiding cow's milk doesn't need to mean missing out. Replace cow's milk with almond milk, coconut milk or rice milk. Replace cow's cheese with goat's and sheep's cheese. You can get goat's yoghurt, nut and seed butters, have dark chocolate instead of milk chocolate. Goat's and sheep's dairy is easier to digest, does not have all the added hormones, has fewer allergenic proteins, causes less inflammation and is higher in calcium as well, so we can absorb it better.

#9
YOUR CORE IS USED WITH EVERY EXERCISE.

In the Viking Method there are no core crunches, no fast core bicycles or throwing your legs aimlessly up and down. The core is worked as the centre of your body, the connector and the glue that keeps you together. You will not be going through your programme and only focusing on your core for the last 5 minutes. You will use it in every exercise. Your core is your powerhouse (see box).

The first thing you always need to do is engage your core, and in order to force you to focus on it, the Viking Method is filled with balancing, stability, lateral movement, kicking and explosive exercises. Using your core this way will make it extremely strong; not only that, it will improve your performance in every way. You will run faster, jump higher, stand taller, and tasks in daily life will be easier. You will be tighter, more together; your whole posture and the way you move will be completely different. You will become one of those crazy people that goes up to their friends and says, 'Punch me in the stomach.' And you won't even feel it. (Don't try this at home!)

KNOW YOUR CORE

Your core is comprised of layers of muscle around your midline (front and back) which support your pelvis and spine. These muscles work as a team to keep your posture in alignment and your back safe from any strain or unwanted force that might cause pain or injury down the road.

Your core acts as a movement ignitor, a dynamic or static stabilizer, and also moves force from one extremity to another. The use of your core is present in all three planes of movement – it is highly functional. Most of the time, your core is much more of a stabilizer and a massive centre for force transference than the actual isolated prime mover.

But still, most people work it as an isolated identity, for example by doing core crunches. When you train it that way, you are missing out not only on a huge part of the core's function but also on improvement in power, agility, strength, better movement in general, as well as longevity in greater health.

In the Viking Method we train the core as it is designed to be trained. As a powerhouse, as a bringer of force, as a 'solid as an oak' stabilizer. Vikings consciously use it in every single exercise. Because it is used in every single exercise!

Get ready to be an absolute Core Slayer!

#10
NO BEFORE AND AFTER PHOTOGRAPHS.

'Before and after' photographs are definitely not a true indicator of your progress. That is why in the Viking Method we do 'before and after' performances, AKA the Viking Challenge.

On the first day of your programme you do a specific Viking Challenge for a certain length of time and note how many reps you did. Then you do your programme, and on the last day you repeat the Challenge.

Doing the Challenge again, and seeing how much more you can achieve, is amazing. It gives you such a feeling of accomplishment to realize you can do so much more than you thought you were capable of. Photographs do not show this change, and they carry with them such inherent negativity. You might be happy for a second but then you'll start seeing all the things that you think still need changing. There is always some other 'flaw' that needs improvement, there is always someone that you feel has a better body than you have now, which means that you will always need validation from others. This is why we are putting the focus on what you do. This is where you always win. And I promise you, it will change you forever. See the Viking Challenge on page 32 to join in the action!

#11
ALWAYS PREPARE.

Preparation is crucial. Know what you are going to eat, know what you are going to do when you train and know what your goals are.

Plan all your meals in advance: this makes it so much easier to make healthy choices rather than snap decisions when you're already hungry. Prepare your 'out' meals (work lunches and so on) either 3 days in advance (you can leave any cooked food in the fridge for 3 days) or the night before, when you are cooking dinner.

Always have a training plan. Never start your session without knowing what you are going to do. Otherwise it is very difficult to last through hard sets and not give up: having certain exercises that you have to finish before you can stop pushes you on.

#12
WE DO WHAT IS HARD, SO OUR LIFE WILL BE EASY.

If you grab life by the horns, demand more from yourself and others, don't take no for an answer, stand by your beliefs and know that you are willing to do whatever it takes, then you will succeed. Yes, it is hard, but it is worth it. Most importantly, you are worth it. Because if you put the hard work in now, your life will be easy. The Viking training changes your mindset. It makes you see that you are not weak. That you are not timid or limited. It makes you realize just how capable, how mighty, how authoritative you really are. It helps you to make your life easier.

THINK
LIKE A VIKING

Being a Viking has nothing to do with where you are from. It has nothing to do with anything outside of you.

Being a Viking represents a certain way of thinking, of doing, of being. It is all about who you choose to be.

Being a Viking is always knowing that the quality of your life is up to you. It's knowing that what you do is what you get. Who you work on being is who you will become.

From now on, in everything you do, whether it's your training, your work or your social life, channel your inner Viking by applying these principles:

» VIKINGS TAKE FULL RESPONSIBILITY FOR THEMSELVES AND THEIR LIVES

You need to stop blaming other people and situations for where you are now. As long as you do that, you will stay in that place because you cannot change what somebody else does, you can only change what you do. As soon as you take responsibility and accept that you are where you are now because of your choices, your actions and your inactions, you have taken your power back. Take the reins by taking the responsibility.

» VIKINGS KNOW WHAT THEY WANT

What do *you* want? In every aspect of your life you need to know deeply, consciously, without a shadow of a doubt what you want, because if you do not know what you want, you cannot do anything to bring yourself closer to achieving your goal. If you do not know what you want, you will wake up every day and have to take whatever life throws at you. Therefore, first and foremost, you need to decide what you want.

What do you want from your career? What do you want from your physical state? What do you want from your nutrition? What do you want from your personal life? What do you want from yourself? Decide, write it down, and then you can do something about it.

» VIKINGS HAVE STAMINA

When you know what you want, then it's time to activate your stamina to work to get it. I am not talking about treadmill stamina. I am talking about mental stamina.

Building up your mental stamina means that at the first sign of something getting a little bit tough, you don't just give up and go back to excuses and blaming others. If you want it to be all about easy, then stay in that discontented place. It's easy to stay unhappy and complain about it but do nothing to change it.

Start now by aligning your actions with your desires and with what you say you want. You have the stamina for this. And with every workout you finish, with every increased level of your physical stamina, you will build up your mental stamina. Your workouts will prove to your mind that you've got this.

» VIKINGS ARE NOT OK WITH NOT BEING OK

If you want to change your reality, you need to change what you are doing. If you are in a place that you are unhappy with and you want to take yourself to a new, better place, then you cannot keep on doing the same actions, and inactions, that you have been doing and getting really surprised that nothing changes.

It's like if I wanted to go to Paris but kept on boarding a plane to Barcelona, then, every time I landed in Barcelona, I was really surprised that I was not in Paris once again.

Stop being so OK with not being OK and make a change.

VIKING MANTRA #4
NOBODY IS COMING TO FIX THINGS FOR YOU. THIS IS YOUR LIFE. FIX IT YOUR VIKING SELF.

» VIKINGS ARE NOT FEELERS

You have taken responsibility. You know what you want. You have stamina. Now don't let your feelings mess it up. Own your feelings and learn to control them. You are not your feelings. Don't be a person who gives up because they don't feel like it.

'I don't *feel* like getting up at 5.30 a.m.'
'I don't *feel* like working on my business on a Friday night.'
'I don't *feel* like exercising on a Sunday.'

Do you think people who get to the top only do what they feel like? No – they do what they need to do to achieve their goals no matter what they feel like. Because they know that it will always be worth it in the long run.

Don't let your feelings stop you. You have a goal, a vision, a dream: go after it fully. No matter what you feel like.

» VIKINGS ARE PRECIOUS ABOUT THEIR TIME

Be very precious about your time: it goes by so quickly. Don't waste it in a job or a relationship that doesn't make you happy. We often equate longevity with quality or success: 'If I have been doing something for a long time, it must mean it's working.' No, it just means you have been doing it for a long time.

Holding on to something simply for the sake of holding on to it does not make it a success. There is no prize or trophy for 'hanging in there'.

Leaving something that gives you no growth, no stimulation and no happiness does not mean that you are giving up. Settling, staying: those things mean giving up.

» VIKINGS DO NOT STAY IN THE PAST

The past belongs in the past. Yes, we all have gone through some rough times and gone through failures, but you have to stop dragging yours around with you.

Just because things might not have worked out then, does not mean they won't now. The only thing you will achieve by keeping the past with you is prevent yourself from achieving your goals in the present and the future.

So don't walk into a new relationship being extremely hard on your new partner because your last partner was an absolute asshole. Or hold off on improving your health because the last time you tried you gave up, so what's the point of trying again?

Ask yourself these questions:

❯ What am I prepared to do now to make this change happen, that I didn't do then?

❯ What can I do better than last time?

Find the answers and apply them. It's all about changing your approach – only then will you get a different outcome.

» VIKINGS GO TO BED IN PEACE

We have got so used to needing approval and validation from others that we have stopped going: 'Hang on, what do I think of this? Does this fit within my value system?'

I cannot tell you how many meetings I have been to about the future of my company and with people who want to collaborate with me where they say: 'OK, let's start doing before and after pictures and more bikini shots of you in the gym, because financially that will grow it quickly.'

I always tell them that's not what my company is about or who I am. And no matter what the gains may be, I will never compromise on my values.

At the end of each day, I want to be able to sleep in peace. I want to be fine with myself, with who I am. And if I do something that's not true to me, I wouldn't be able to do that.

This goes for your personal life too. If there's somebody in your life who makes you feel like you have to dismiss who you are and your value system in order to keep them, they are not worth keeping.

Never trade your integrity for an opportunity. Always go to bed being at peace with who you are.

>> VIKINGS ALWAYS KNOW THEIR WORTH

You determine your own worth, not other people. Whatever behaviour you accept, both from other people and from yourself, is the kind of behaviour that you will continue to receive. Know that being a loving, kind, caring person definitely does not mean allowing people to treat you however they want. You are not a football to be kicked around.

If your closest company does not add to you – if they do not support you, if they do not stimulate you, if they do not treat you with love and respect – then it's time for you to find new company that values you as much as you value yourself.

If you have to say things like, 'Deep down he/she is good' or, 'Deep down he/she loves me,' then trust me, that person isn't good enough for you. You should never have to dig for goodness or for love.

Stop adjusting yourself to suit someone else. Stop dumbing yourself down, devaluing who

you are. You should never contain yourself for the comfort of others. You should never suppress your voice or your immense being in order not to rock the boat. Rock that longboat!

>> VIKINGS LACK NOTHING

One of the questions I get asked most often is: 'If I go to the gym five times a week and eat really healthily, how long will it take for me to look like *them*?' The answer is: never.

You are not that person. You are put together in a different way. Stop comparing yourself to others and believing that you lack something. For example, I am very straight: I do not have much of a waist and no matter what I do, I will never have a tiny waist. Therefore, if I think that I do not look good unless I have a small waist and try everything to get that, I am screwed. I will always be unhappy with the way I look, because that is just not the body I have. I will see women with small waists and feel that I lack that. But if I stop comparing myself to others, and just focus on making me as great as I can be, then I am unbreakable.

Do not start anything from a place of lacking. You lack nothing. By training and eating healthily you are only adding to yourself. I read about this great survey where grown-ups and kids were asked: 'If you could change anything about yourself, what would you change?' All the grown-ups wanted to take something away. They said things like: 'I would like a different nose', 'smaller thighs' or 'a bigger bum'. All the kids wanted to add something: 'I would like to have massive wings', 'a bottomless stomach so I can eat loads' or 'a tail'. None of the kids thought that they needed to replace anything about themselves. By following the Viking Method you are adding to how great you already are. Time to grow some massive grown-up wings!

YOUR HORMONES

The idea that changing your body shape is all to do with calories in vs. calories out is outdated and just not right. Yes, we need to watch that we do not eat too much, but we have to understand that consuming 1500 kcal in Mars Bars will have a totally different effect from eating 1500 kcal in fish, chicken, vegetables and fibrous fruit. What is important is where your energy (aka calories) is coming from and how that affects your body, and your hormones in particular.

The role of your hormones is crucial and vast: they control the rates of certain chemical reactions, assist in transporting substances through membranes, and help regulate water balance, electrolyte balance (electrolytes are substances that create an electric charge and that are essential for numerous bodily functions) and blood pressure. They manage development, growth, reproduction and behaviour. They are the body's messengers, which get produced in one part of the body such as the thyroid or the adrenal glands, pass into the bloodstream or other body fluid, and go to distant organs and tissues where they act to modify structures and functions. They are like traffic signals, telling our body what to do and when, so it can run smoothly and efficiently. Your hormones control lean tissue building, ageing, your fight or flight response, your energy burning and your metabolic rate. Understanding how they work and, in turn, what makes them work is necessary for optimum health.

Out of these amazing amounts of hormones you have six fat-burning hormones (such as the growth hormone) and three fat-storing hormones (such as insulin). These two groups cannot be fully activated at the same time, which means that when one fat-storing hormone is activated it will de-activate all your fat-burning hormones. The fat-burning hormones are also anti-ageing, de-stressing and lean tissue-building.

In the Viking Method we train and eat to activate the fat-burning hormones, not the fat-storing hormones.

TRAINING FOR YOUR HORMONES

BEFORE TRAINING

When you train, you want to activate your fat-burning hormones. In order for that to happen, certain things must be done. If you have sugar before training, you activate insulin (fat-storing), which will stop the fat-burning hormones working properly while you exercise. Therefore, do not have any carbohydrates for 90 minutes before you train. I am not saying train hungry, I'm just saying you should time your foods and think ahead.

DURING TRAINING

After warming up, in order to activate the growth hormone (the fat-burning, anti-ageing, lean tissue-building hormone), you need to do high-intensity training, i.e. training that is all out for short periods but with breaks in between, like sprints on the treadmill (30 seconds on, 1 minute off). You will need the breaks, because you can't keep up the high-intensity level that is needed for long periods. Also, exercise puts stress on the body and that stress, over a prolonged period, will activate cortisol (a fat-storing hormone). The breaks are just as important in this kind of training as the exercise. The growth hormone can only be activated through high-intensity training. You should be training so hard that you cannot still hold a conversation.

AFTER TRAINING

Often, no matter how hard you train, there will be a stubborn area on your body; an area where you feel you just cannot get rid of the fat. For many women it is the hips and bum, and for men the stomach (but it can be other areas as well, of course). There is a scientific reason behind this. On every fat cell there are two receptors called Alpha and Beta receptors. The Alpha generates fat-storing and has little blood flow; the Beta generates fat-burning and is rich in blood flow. In these stubborn areas, there are many more Alpha receptors than Beta, which is why it is that much harder to get rid of the fat.

In order to tackle this fat a few things need to happen. Due to the low blood flow in these areas, after your high-intensity training you need to keep the blood flow up so the body is able to transfer the fat to places where it will get burned. Therefore, **after you have done your Viking programme, you should always do a 10-minute jog**. Nothing fast, just enough to keep you warm and your blood flowing. Alternatively, you could do a yoga flow, or put your favourite song on and dance. You choose: just keep moving.

EATING FOR YOUR HORMONES

THE GROWTH HORMONE

The growth hormone is highly activated during the first hour after you fall asleep. That's the high time where your body is restoring itself. So here is another 90-minute rule: **No carbs 90 minutes before you go to bed.**

Carbohydrates before bed will disrupt the activation of the growth hormone and other hormones that are taking good care of you. The only time this rule gets overwritten is if you happen to train right before bed, in which case you need to eat carbs afterwards, even if it is closer than 90 minutes to bedtime.

Focus your carbohydrate intake mostly on vegetables and fibrous fruit. If you are a person who craves carbs such as rice, pasta, bread, then have your Sometimes Carbs right after you train (along with protein and/or fat), as your muscles will be screaming for energy and it will go straight into feeding them instead of hanging around in your bloodstream and being stored as fat.

You always need to have Sometimes Carbs after you train. Your muscles need that refuelling to be ready for the next workout. See post-training recipes (pages 118–57).

GHRELIN

Ghrelin is produced in the stomach and tends to rise before meals and fall after them. It is called the 'hunger hormone', because it is the appetite-stimulating hormone in humans and is the contributing factor in giving people cravings for unhealthy snacks.

Ghrelin is also released in response to stressful situations, which is why many people have the tendency to eat when they are stressed. By being in a cycle of constant stress, ghrelin contributes to weight gain by maintaining a person's stress levels and giving that person the urge to eat unhealthily. As well as stress, sleep deprivation has been shown to produce an increase in ghrelin.

LEPTIN

Leptin is the antagonist hormone. It is referred to as the 'starvation hormone', as it sends a signal to the brain that you have enough food in your stomach and your energy levels are sufficient. The body produces leptin based on your fat percentage levels. Weight gain will cause a rise in your leptin and, in theory, weight loss should then happen. But when you are overweight or obese, you become leptin-resistant, meaning that your leptin signals do not properly reach your brain, resulting in further weight gain as you require more food to 'feel' full.

When you start doing your Viking programme, your fat percentage will go down, your internal stress will decrease and you will start to sleep better, bringing these hormones to balance, which will make them work for you, not against you.

LOOK AFTER YOUR LIVER

Good liver function is crucial, as many of your fat-burning hormones are metabolized by the liver. Therefore you need to take care of it:

› Have plenty of greens: green vegetables, green salads, spirulina.

› Reduce your coffee and alcohol consumption – Vikings like a beer, but try to indulge only occasionally.

› Have healthy fats, e.g. avocados, nuts, coconut oil, fish oils.

› Drink plenty of water – aim for between 1.2 and 2 litres a day.

› Stay clear of junk food and trans fats (see Eat Like a Viking, pages 91–2, for more on different types of fat).

› Exercise: five times a week; two high-intensity functional programmes that you repeat, where you are using both your body weight and free weights, and one Madness programme. Basically, do the Viking Method training!

› Buy organic produce where possible, to remove toxins and pesticides from your diet.

VIKING MANTRA #5

YOU WILL ALWAYS BE TOO MUCH OF SOMETHING FOR SOMEONE: TOO BIG, TOO LOUD, TOO SMART OR TOO STRONG. WHEN THAT HAPPENS, IT IS UP TO THAT PERSON TO DEAL WITH IT. NOT YOU. APOLOGIZE FOR MISTAKES. APOLOGIZE FOR UNINTENTIONALLY HURTING SOMEBODY. BUT DO NOT APOLOGIZE FOR WHO YOU ARE. NEVER BE EASY. NEVER BE EASILY MANIPULATED, BOUGHT, INFLUENCED OR DEFEATED. THE ONLY APPROVAL YOU EVER NEED IS YOUR OWN. STAND YOUR GROUND.

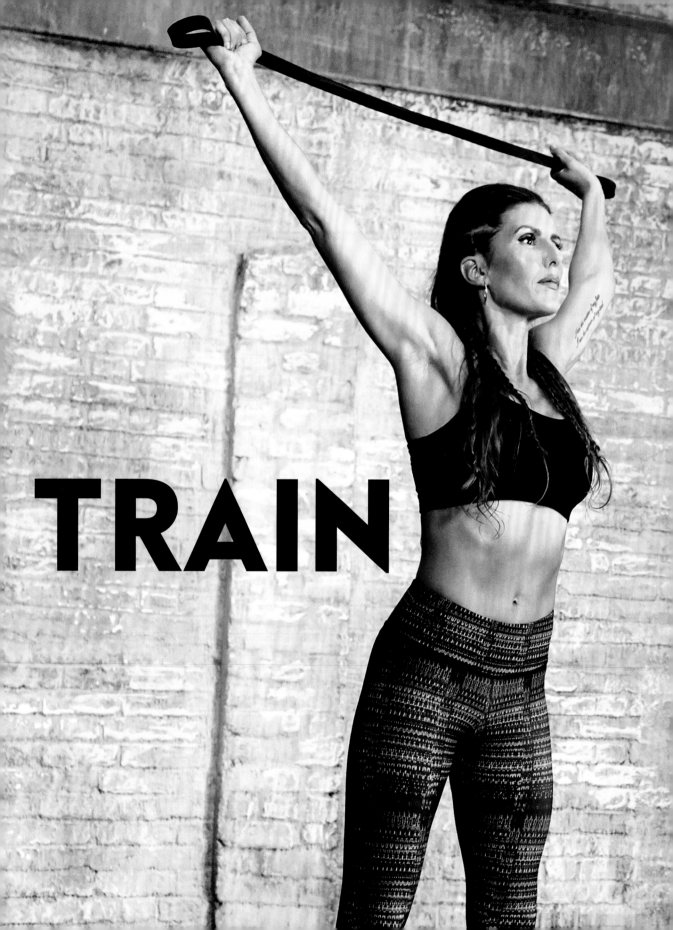

TRAIN

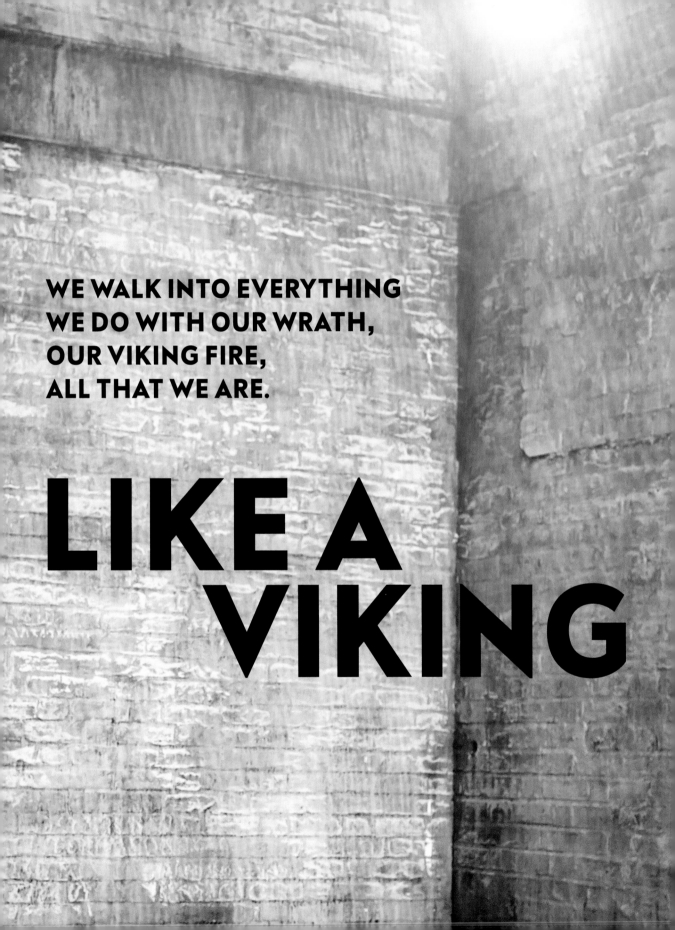

WE WALK INTO EVERYTHING
WE DO WITH OUR WRATH,
OUR VIKING FIRE,
ALL THAT WE ARE.

LIKE A VIKING

VIKING MANTRA #6

DON'T LET THERE BE A MUSCLE IN YOUR BODY WITHOUT A GREAT PURPOSE.
DON'T LET THE ONLY FUNCTION OF YOUR BODY BE EXTERNAL APPEARANCE.
YOUR BODY, YOUR BRAIN AND YOUR HEART ARE ALL UNBELIEVABLE TOOLS WITH INFINITE POSSIBILITIES. USE THEM TO THE FULLEST.
PHYSICALLY TRAIN FOR MAXIMUM CAPABILITY. TRAIN YOUR BODY TO BE UNBREAKABLE, TO BE QUICK, STRONG, FLEXIBLE AND POWERFUL.
TAKE UP A NEW SKILL: LEARN TO PLAY AN INSTRUMENT, LEARN A NEW LANGUAGE, TO PAINT OR TO KNIT. OPEN YOURSELF TO NEW EXPERIENCES, PEOPLE AND OPPORTUNITIES.
GIVE MORE OF YOURSELF. MAKE A FOOL OF YOURSELF. FAIL. GO AGAIN. HUG THE PEOPLE AROUND YOU. LAUGH OUT LOUD OFTEN. COMPLIMENT A STRANGER. BE KIND.
GIVE YOURSELF GREAT PURPOSE.

» VIKINGS TRAIN WITHOUT MACHINES

We use free weights and our own body weight: crawling, pushing, pulling, rotating, kicking – huge amounts of plyometric exercises. Plyometric means 'jump training' – exercises where we make the muscles use maximum force in short intervals to increase power and speed.

» VIKINGS FOCUS ON THE FAST-TWITCH MUSCLE FIBRES

These are the muscles that are the most powerful but that fatigue quickly. There are different types of muscle fibres in the body, generally categorized into slow-twitch and fast-twitch muscle fibres. The fast-twitch are the explosive, the strong, the powerful ones. And we work them. We slay them.

» VIKINGS DO SPECIFIC EXERCISES THAT WE PAIR IN A CERTAIN WAY

Typically this might mean a high-intensity functional exercise (e.g. burpees, see page 67) followed by a more static functional exercise (e.g. press-ups, see page 49), done within a certain time frame or a certain amount of reps. This forces you to utilize more energy and oxygen and at the same time create more lean tissue as well as activate the growth hormone, the king hormone of fat-burning. Training like this creates an after-burn that is very beneficial as it raises your metabolic rate, meaning you will continue to burn more energy long after you stop training. In order to keep this higher rate up, never go longer than 48 hours between sessions, as after that time your metabolic rate will start to drop.

» VIKINGS TRAIN UNTIL THEY ARE UNCOMFORTABLE

Nothing is easy. Your body doesn't like change and therefore you will have to force the change – you need to push it. So, be uncomfortable. If the last few reps or the last few seconds are not a complete struggle, you are not working hard enough and you will not see any change. If you are a normally healthy person, make use of it. Push yourself. Value your time and the body you have. No matter how fit or unfit you are, you should always be completely exhausted at the end of your workout. No more faffing about and then being upset that you are not seeing much change. Expect more from yourself and you will start to reap more.

» VIKINGS DO NOT WEIGH THEMSELVES

Being obsessed with how much you weigh is a waste of your energy and says nothing about your progression. Muscle weighs more than fat and takes up less space. Therefore, you could weigh the same, or heaven forbid even more, and be leaner and fitter, with a lower fat percentage. Throw out the scales.

This is it, Viking. This is the time, the time when you decide that you are done with giving in, giving up and not giving it your all.

This is the time when *you* say:
I DARE. I CAN. I WILL.

Now get ready to go berserk.

THE VIKING CHALLENGE

VIKING MANTRA #7

START ALIGNING YOUR ACTIONS WITH YOUR DESIRES AND WHAT YOU SAY YOU WANT. STOP BEING COMFORTABLE WITH SITTING ON A NAIL AND CONTINUOUSLY COMPLAINING ABOUT THE PAIN OF THE NAIL. GET OFF THE NAIL.

OUR BEFORE AND AFTER

The Viking Challenge is one of the foundations of the Viking Method. The purpose of the Challenge is for you to see the impact of all that you have achieved since beginning the Viking Method and really feel the difference the additional strength, mental force and energy that you have built up has made.

Bookending your Four Weeks of Wrath is Loki's Challenge.

Loki is the trickster God. The most dangerous deity in Norse mythology, he is a shape-shifter and an extremely clever and immensely powerful magician. Channel his magic in this challenge!

Loki's Challenge is simple: count how many burpees you can do in 5 minutes. It doesn't matter if you need to take a long break or more than one break – as long as you're doing the very best you can, then that's enough. The only thing you need is a timer and every last bit of your Viking willpower.

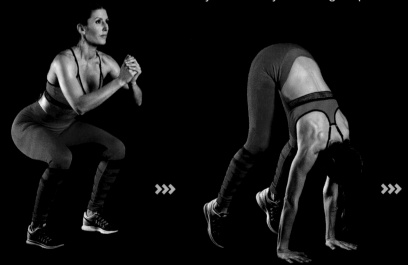

A burpee is an exercise that works your entire body. Here's how to do one:

1 Squat with your bum going back, and place your hands down on the floor between your legs.

2 Jump backwards into a press-up position (do not bring your chest down to the floor).

3 Jump back to the squat, jump up explosively with your hands coming above your head, and land in a squat. That is one burpee.

Tip: The main thing to watch, and this is crucial, is that when you jump out of the press-up position back into the squat, your heels need to be down on the ground. Keep your shoulders back, torso straight and engage your core!

When you do the challenge at the start, do not analyse or judge your performance. This is the 'before' performance, so of course there is going to be room for improvement: don't be negative about it. Just do as many burpees as you can – don't stop until the timer goes; yes, have a breather within that time if you need to and as many as you need to, but then always keep on going. Do not quit before the time is up. Then write your reps down when you're finished, and get ready to start slaying your month.

Really try your hardest, and don't give up. If the idea of giving up enters your head, pay it no attention. You will finish these 5 minutes no matter what.

After a month of training, do the challenge again. You will marvel at the progress you've made and it will be impossible to be negative about how much stronger and more determined you've become.

You can smash this. Let's do it!

BEFORE: . . . Burpees . . . Reps:

AFTER: . . . Burpees . . . Reps:

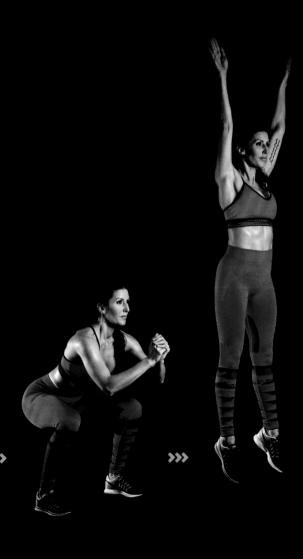

FOUR WEEKS OF WRATH

THE IMPORTANCE OF KNOWLEDGE IN THE VIKING TRAINING

VIKINGS HAVE A POWERHOUSE CORE

Being conscious of your core, engaging it, and working it properly will not only make it stronger, but will also help you to perform the exercises correctly, make you more powerful, and greatly enhance your performance as well as your posture and ability to carry out everyday tasks.

Now, engaging your core is a completely different thing from sucking in your stomach. When you engage your core, it should make you feel very rooted and secure. You feel strong and stable.

1 Roll your shoulders back so that your chest appears tall and proud.

2 Keep your ribs from flaring outwards: stack them right under your chest. Your lower back should be long.

3 Gently tuck your pelvis under and fire your glute muscles (bum muscles) and you should start to feel your core engage.

4 Imagine that you are bracing yourself for a hard punch in the stomach. Now you should really feel your core!

Transverse abdominis (TVA) is the deepest of the four muscle groups that make up the abdominals (the others are rectus abdominis, the external obliques, and the internal obliques). The muscle acts like a girdle and plays an important role in spinal stability.

To feel your TVA, lie on your back on the floor with your knees bent and legs relaxed.

1 Place the fingers of your left hand on your left hipbone. Move them 8 centimetres sideways towards the centre line of your body and then 2 centimetres down.

2 Tuck your pelvis under and start engaging your core.

3 Press your fingers slightly into your body. Then try to press against your fingers from within! You will feel a deep-rooted pressure against them pressing them back out. That is your TVA.

VIKINGS HAVE GREAT MOTOR SKILLS

'Motor skills' refers to the ability to perform complex muscular acts that produce movement, achieved through communication and coordination between the brain, nervous system and muscles.

One big way to improve your motor skills is by respecting every single exercise and every single part of every single exercise. Don't perform them half-heartedly. Don't let your mind wander to the past or future, and don't move without engagement and precision. If you do, then when you finish training you might say, 'I didn't feel it that much.' Of course you didn't, you weren't really there when you were doing it. Be there fully. Don't waste your time. Get the most out of every exercise. Always feel it that much.

Every movement starts in the mind, and intention creates action.

When you train you need to be fully present. Each and every movement needs to be performed with purpose and focus. Just going through the motions while thinking about something else (or thinking 'God, this is hard'), will give you completely different results from if you clear your mind, and really feel your energy, breathing deeply and thinking: 'I am going to lift this weight,' or, 'I am going to root my heels down, engage my core, squeeze my glutes and I will not stop until I have finished.'

Vikings are always present. And that is why they have the skills. Because they have worked for them.

VIKINGS ARE MASTERS OF BALANCE

Training in the Viking Method places great importance on increasing your balance, and this is why:

❯ Balancing exercises benefit your neuromuscular coordination, strengthen your joints and ligaments, and place a different stressor on your working muscle, therefore making it more powerful, helping with hip stabilization, and improving your core strength.

❯ Good balance makes it much easier to stay cool, calm and collected when your longboat hits a storm.

SUN'S OUT, VIKINGS ARE OUT!

There are so many benefits to training outside: getting that dose of vitamin D, expending more energy (the body needs to work doubly hard, as it is constantly cooling you down), not to mention the extreme mental boost. Nature has such a de-stressing, calming effect and at the same time it energizes and revitalizes you, leading to a greater release of your happy hormones and a higher intake of oxygen. So when the sun is out, the Vikings are out slaying it (with sunscreen of course).

KNOWLEDGE IS POWER BUT ONLY IF YOU APPLY ACTION TO IT. APPLY EVERYTHING THAT FOLLOWS TO YOUR TRAINING.

VIKING MANTRA #8

NEVER DO ANYTHING JUST TO PROVE SOMEBODY ELSE WRONG. DO NOT MAKE WHAT YOU DO ABOUT SOMEBODY ELSE. THIS IS ABOUT YOU. THIS IS YOUR CHANGE. THEREFORE, WHATEVER YOU DO, ALWAYS DO IT TO PROVE YOURSELF RIGHT.

VIKINGS ALWAYS WARM UP

Your body needs to warm up so that you will not injure yourself, so that your systems get ready for the workout, start increasing oxygen and blood flow into your muscles, limber your joints up and get you mentally prepared for the berserkness ahead.

Always warm up for 5 minutes before you start, whether it's jogging, cycling, lifting your knees high on the spot, skipping, or dancing to your favourite songs.

Then do gentle exercises for 5 minutes: slow squats, one-legged squats touching your hands down to the floor, walk-downs to a high plank position (see page 41) and back up, one-legged swinging your leg up forward and backward, standing straight and twisting your torso sideways, and running your knees in towards your chest in a high plank position.

Do not do any static stretching before you train, such as bending over to touch your toes, standing on one leg and bending the other leg with the heel of the foot to your bum, or stretching your hamstrings by placing your leg on a bench and leaning over. Stretching before training can actually cause your muscles to tighten rather than relax, and you are more likely to pull a muscle. It's like extending a rubber band to its limits, making it more likely to snap.

VIKINGS ALWAYS COOL DOWN

After you finish your training, cool down for 5–10 minutes (fast walking, jogging, moving on the spot, skipping, dancing – anything!). The cool-down is very important for your stubborn fat areas, as you need to keep the blood flow up after finishing your high-intensity training.

Vikings end their session with stretching too. A good range of motion is needed to swing that sword around!

When you are done with the warm-up, the slaying and the cool-down, it's time for your static stretching.

Stretching after training reduces muscle tension as well as aiding in muscle recovery and repair. Stretching also improves range of motion, increases muscular coordination, and increases your flexibility, which prevents injuries, betters your posture and enhances your performance and everyday movements.

On the days when you are doing your Viking Madness (see pages 58–63), allow more time for stretching: the Madness takes less time than the programmes – instead spend the extra time properly stretching your whole body. Hold each stretch for 30–60 seconds. No pulsing, just gently increasing the stretch throughout. Use your breath – with every outbreath, you should go a little deeper into the stretch.

See pages 84–7 for more on Post Cool-down Stretches.

THE PROGRAMME

There are so many shortcuts in life that we can take now, that we get surprised when the 3-minute ab crunch workout didn't give us the visible 6-pack we wanted, or that we have gained back the weight we lost during the 2-week water and syrup diet.

It's because you are trying to take shortcuts where there isn't a shortcut available. Minimum work gives minimum, short-lived results. The Viking Method is about life-changing, long-lasting, maximum results.

» **Each week** you have two high-intensity functional programmes and one Viking Madness. With warm-up, cool-down and stretching, each programme should take around 35–40 minutes in total.

» **Every week** you do each programme twice and the Madness once. Weeks 1 and 2 are the same. Weeks 3 and 4 are the same. The Viking Madness stays the same throughout the month.

» It is better for the body to **repeat programmes** for a certain amount of time to enable yourself to get better at them, master the technique, and really up your power and stamina each time. Then, when you have them down, you switch it up!

THE VIKING EQUIPMENT THAT YOU NEED:

» A skipping rope.

» An exercise mat.

» Two tea towels or exercise gliders (if you're training on a carpet rather than a smooth-surfaced floor, you can use a couple of magazines).

» One/two sets of dumbbells (ideally one lighter and one heavier, but just one set is also fine). The dumbbells should be at a weight where the final three reps of the exercise that you are doing are a struggle. If you feel the same doing the last rep as you felt when you did the first rep, then the weights are too light. Remember: it's always about being comfortable with being uncomfortable!

PROGRAMME BASICS

Each programme is made up of:

» Two groups of three exercises in a row.

» Four sets of each group.

» A 45-second rest between sets.

» A 2-minute rest before moving on to the next group of exercises.

EXAMPLE: VIKING PLAN OF ATTACK

	Mon	Tues	Weds	Thurs	Fri	Sat	Sun
Week 1	Programme 1	Programme 2	Rest	Programme 1	Programme 2	Madness	Rest
Week 2	Programme 1	Programme 2	Rest	Programme 1	Programme 2	Madness	Rest
Week 3	Programme 3	Programme 4	Rest	Programme 3	Programme 4	Madness	Rest
Week 4	Programme 3	Programme 4	Rest	Programme 3	Programme 4	Madness	Rest

Write down your reps for the Before and After Challenge and your weekly time for the Madness. You have space for this underneath your Weekly Viking Training and Nutrition Plan on page 230.

DON'T FORGET TO DO YOUR VIKING CHALLENGE BEFORE YOU BEGIN, AND AGAIN AT THE END OF THE 4 WEEKS!

THE THREE FUNDAMENTAL VIKING TRAINING POSITIONS

These positions are used continuously throughout the Viking training and they are all extremely powerful. Therefore, I have given each one a name that represents them and what you should be channelling, both physically and mentally, when you carry them out – in return, these are the benefits you will get back, multiplied.

You never just 'do' these, or any other positions or exercises in the Viking Method. You bring everything you are and all of yourself into each one. You engage every muscle, every ounce of focus you have, and every part of you is fully present.

#1
THE READY FOR BATTLE STANCE POSITION

Stand tall, head held high, shoulders back, core engaged, feet hip width apart, feet and knees facing forward with 'ready to slay' energy running through your body! Feel the courage that you possess, the persistence, the resilience. Know that you will be victorious.

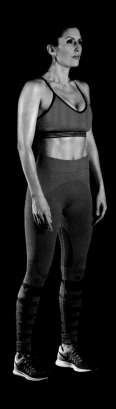

#2
THE ENERGY SQUAT POSITION

Start in Battle Stance. Sit back and down like you are sitting on an imaginary stool that is far behind you. Heels are rooted into the ground, knees are bent and straight over toes. Upper body bends forward a bit but your back is straight and your chest is up. You are deep in that energy position, with your hip crease going past your knees. Engage your core, feel every muscle working in your body. Your arms are in front of you, bent at the elbow.

#3
THE ROOT POWER HIGH PLANK POSITION

Come down to the floor on all fours, positioning your hands straight under your shoulders (wrists in line with shoulders). Extend your legs back, hip width apart so you are balancing on your hands and feet. Keep your arms straight and your shoulders down, not letting them move up to your ears. Keep a straight line from the top of your head all the way down to your heels. Tuck your pelvis under, keeping your lower back long and your core fully engaged. Feel the power from the earth flowing into your body through your hands and feet. You are well rooted and secure.

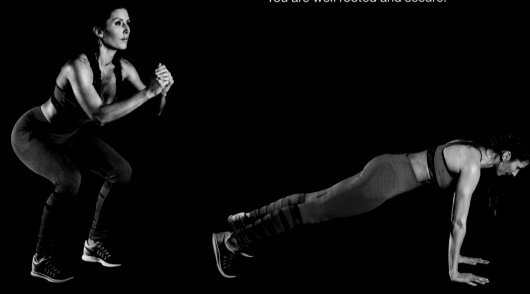

NOW, LET'S START THE PROGRAMME! IT'S TIME TO GO BERSERK.

WEEKS 1 & 2
PROGRAMME 1

GROUP 1

EXERCISES 1, 2, 3 IN A ROW.
FOUR SETS.
45-SECOND REST BETWEEN SETS.
2-MINUTE REST

GROUP 2

EXERCISES 4, 5, 6 IN A ROW.
FOUR SETS.
45-SECOND REST BETWEEN SETS.

WEEKS 1 & 2
PROGRAMME 1 GROUP 1
THREE EXERCISES IN A ROW. FOUR SETS OF EACH.
45-SECOND REST BETWEEN SETS.

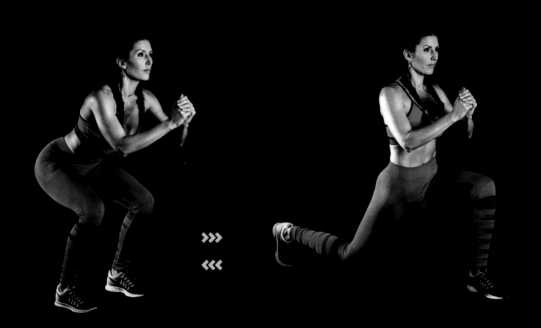

1 SQUAT WITH A BACKWARD LUNGE
30 SECONDS ON EACH LEG

>>> Start in your Energy Squat position (see page 41).

>>> Step your right leg back, bending it, ending in a lunge with the knee of the left leg at a 90° bend and the knee of the right leg just hovering above the floor. Your torso should stay upright, with your shoulders back and core engaged. Then step the right leg forward again, and return to that deep squat position.

>>> Repeat with the right leg for 30 seconds, then do the same with the left leg.

>>> Throughout, you should never extend your body fully upright or straighten out your legs. You bounce continuously between that deep squat position and that backward lunge. Have your arms wherever feels comfortable; I always have them bent at the elbow in front of my heart.

2 WALKING HIGH PLANK
45 SECONDS

>>> Start in your Battle Stance (see page 40). Remember that you are powerful!

>>> Squat down, bringing your arms to the floor and walking your arms forward into the Root Power High Plank position (see page 41). Keep your core engaged so that there is no arching of your lower back, and your spine is in a straight line.

>>> Begin walking your arms back towards your heels until your heels are rooted back to the ground and you are back in a deep squat.

>>> Slowly lengthen all the way up to that Battle Stance. You're not done here. Get straight back down to that squat and push on through. Throughout, focus on keeping your core engaged.

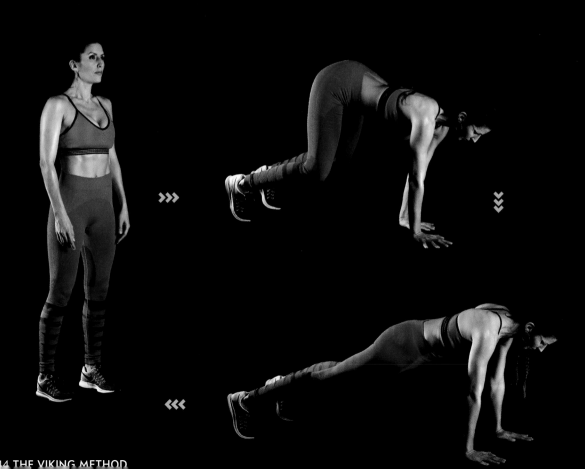

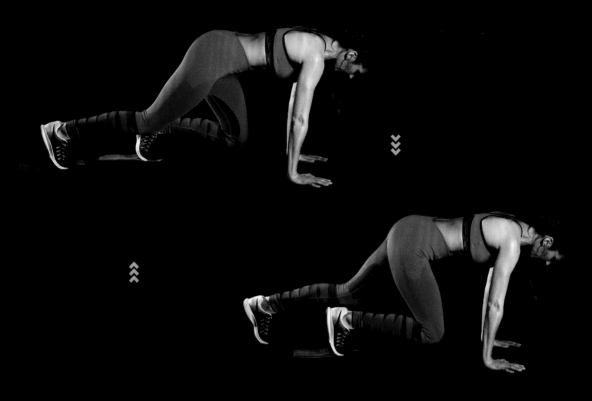

3 RUNNING MAN ON TOWELS
30 SECONDS

>>> Come down into a tabletop position on all fours: your knees on the floor, back straight, palms on the floor with your arms straight (so that your body is in the shape of a table and legs). Have two tea towels or magazines ready and place your toes on top of these. Your wrists should be under your shoulders, your core engaged.

>>> Alternately, run your legs in and out. Don't lift your bum up as you do so and don't place weight on the leg as it comes in, as then you lose the purpose of the exercise. Keep your body in that tabletop position throughout, back in a straight line and arms straight underneath your shoulders. The power of the movement should come from your upper body and core.

>>> Continue for 30 seconds. This is fast – keep at it!

VIKING MENTAL POINTER

WHEN YOU ARE TIRED AND YOUR MIND IS
TRYING TO GET YOU TO GIVE UP, REMEMBER
WHO YOU ARE. YOU ARE NOT WEAK.
THE OPPOSITE: YOU ARE STRONG. YOU
ARE CREATING YOUR OWN CHANGE RIGHT
AT THIS VERY MOMENT BY DOING THIS
PROGRAMME. YOU ARE GIVING UP THINGS
THAT ARE NOT SERVING YOU, AND YOU
ARE ADDING THINGS IN THAT TRULY DO.
EVERYTHING YOU'RE DOING, YOU'VE CHOSEN
TO DO. FOR YOURSELF. BY YOURSELF. FOR
THAT REASON, YOU WILL NOT GIVE UP.
YOU KNOW THAT YOU CAN DO THIS.

1 SQUAT JUMPS 45 SECONDS

>>> Start in your Energy Squat position (see page 41).

>>> Deepen the squat a little bit, then jump up without locking your knees and land back down in that deep, powerful squat.

>>> Power the jump from your hamstrings (the posterior muscles of your upper leg), glutes and core, engaging the muscles. Keep your torso upright and your shoulders down, and make sure that your knees remain in line with your toes as you land – they should stay facing forward and not curve in. Your heels should root to the ground as you land.

>>> Keep on going for 45 seconds.

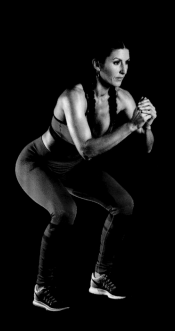

>>>

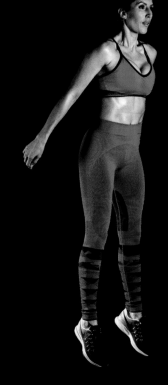

2 SQUAT SHOULDER PRESS
45 SECONDS

>>> Start in your Battle Stance (see page 40). Hold a dumbbell in each hand at shoulder level with the palms facing each other and elbows bent. Remember to keep your elbows tucked in; do not let them flare out.

>>> Push your bottom back, and squat down with your weight going through your heels and backwards (not your knees). Make sure your knees are in line with your toes and not bending inwards. Engage your core muscles and keep your back straight – try not to lean forward.

>>> As you push up through your heels, extend out of the squat and at the same time push your arms up and lengthen them fully over your head, bringing them up into a shoulder press. Engage your glutes (your bum muscles) and your core.

>>> From that highest position, come all the way down into that deep squat again, bringing the arms back down to the shoulders. Remain fast and powerful with your core engaged, as always.

>>> Repeat for 45 seconds.

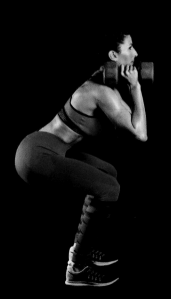
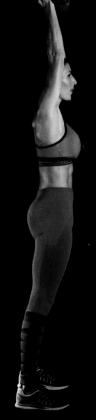

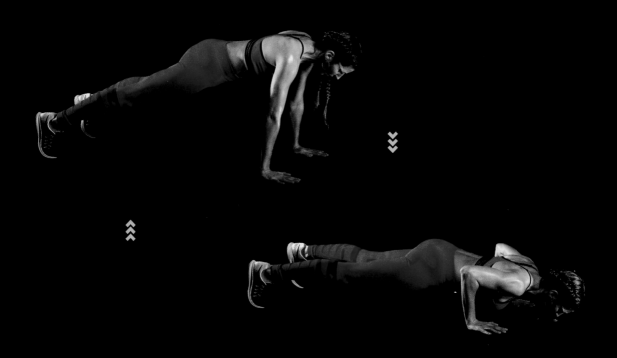

3 **PRESS-UPS** 30 SECONDS

>>> Start in your Root Power High Plank position (see page 41). Now move your hands slightly further apart so that the position of your arms is a bit wider. Remember to tuck your pelvis under and keep your core engaged. Also open up your legs a bit – having them wider will make you use your obliques (side abdominal muscles) more.

>>> Lower your whole body down, until your elbows pass a 90° bend, your chest touches the floor and the rest of your body hovers just above the floor.

>>> Dig deep into that inner strength and push your whole body up in one piece. You should feel this in your chest, arms and stomach muscles, not as an ache in your lower back. If you do, then check your technique, as you are most likely arching your lower back and putting too much pressure on it, which in turn makes it much harder for you to keep your stomach muscles activated. Stop, get your Root Power High Plank position right and keep that long back throughout.

>>> Repeat for 30 seconds.

REMEMBER YOUR POST COOL-DOWN STRETCHES ON PAGES 84–7.

WEEKS 1 & 2
PROGRAMME 2

AFTER YOU HAVE FINISHED ALL THE SETS OF GROUP 1, TAKE A 2-MINUTE REST BEFORE MOVING ON TO GROUP 2 – THIS IS TO CATCH YOUR BREATH AND GET READY FOR THE NEW EXERCISES.

GROUP 1

EXERCISES 1, 2, 3 IN A ROW.
FOUR SETS.
45-SECOND REST BETWEEN SETS.
2-MINUTE REST

GROUP 2

EXERCISES 4, 5, 6 IN A ROW.
FOUR SETS.
45-SECOND REST BETWEEN SETS.

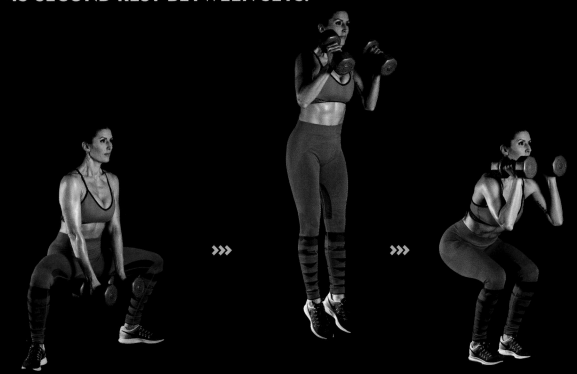

1 WIDE SQUAT TO STRAIGHT SQUAT JUMP WITH BICEP CURL 30 SECONDS

>>> Start in a wide/sumo Energy Squat (wider stance, with legs, knees and feet turned out), holding dumbbells in your hands which should be straight down between your legs with your palms facing each other. Watch that your shoulders do not roll forward and keep your torso straight and chest up.

>>> Jump into a straight squat – your legs, knees and feet should face forward and your legs should be hip width apart – and at the same time engage your biceps (your anterior upper arm muscles), bend your elbows fully up and in towards yourself, ending with your weights in a bicep curl with your palms facing you. There should not be any swing in your arms as you come into the bicep curl – control the movement.

>>> Then jump back into that wide squat with your arms back down between your legs. Focus on getting that wide squat very deep; the straight squat should be less so. Check that your back stays straight throughout and that your heels are rooted into the floor every time you land in those squats.

>>> Repeat for 30 seconds.

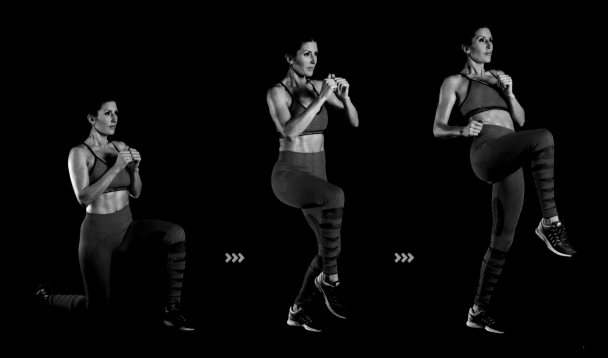

2 KNEELING TO KNEE UP
45 SECONDS ON EACH LEG

>>> Use a mat for this one to protect your knees. Step your left leg far forward and bend the right leg, ending in a deep lunge – so your left leg is bent at a 90° angle and your right leg is bent down with the knee at a 90° angle as well. Keep your torso straight. Now lower that right knee down to the floor, resting the whole of the lower leg on the floor with your foot resting on the floor by its instep. This is your starting position.

>>> Place your weight through your left heel, using your hamstrings and glutes (the posterior muscles in your upper leg and your behind) to come up to standing, bringing your right knee high up in front of you.

>>> Bring that right leg back down to that kneeling position slowly and with a focus on control. Use your core to give you better stability, and keep your shoulders back and back straight. Never use the toes of the back leg to help you to push yourself up. You should only use the front leg. This exercise is all about working your balance, so no cheating!

>>> Repeat for 45 seconds, then change legs and repeat on the other side for 45 seconds. Watch that you don't lean your torso too far forward as you come out of that kneeling position. You want to come straight up. Imagine that you are being pulled straight up from the top of your head.

3 **TRICEP DIPS** 30 SECONDS

⟫⟫ Sit on the edge of a chair or bench and place your hands either side of you on the front edge of the chair close to your bottom. Roll your shoulders back, keeping your lower back long and engaging your core.

⟫⟫ Place your legs slightly further out than 90° (so not in a straight line) with your heels on the floor and your toes lifted up off the floor. Do not place a lot of weight on your heels – your weight should be concentrated through your centre line. Stick your bum out slightly and keep it against the chair – as soon as you come too far out, your legs will take too much of the weight. You shouldn't lean your bum towards your heels – it should sit right underneath that straight back.

⟫⟫ Straighten your arms, keep your back straight, and slowly lower your bottom down towards the floor, keeping your back as close to the chair as possible, so that your weight is in your upper body (working your triceps more – a group of three muscles located at the back of your upper arm) and not moving out into your feet. In that deep position your elbows should be pointing back, and be bent further than 90°.

⟫⟫ Push yourself up using only your triceps. Go as far up as you can without locking the elbows to maintain the tension the whole time.

⟫⟫ Repeat for 30 seconds.

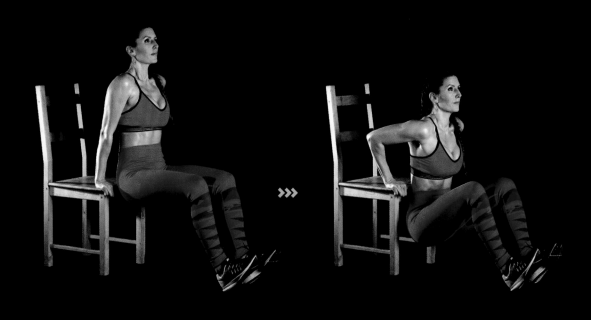

VIKING MENTAL POINTER

WHEN YOU'RE DOING A BALANCE-BASED EXERCISE AND YOU FALL, STOP THINKING, 'I SHOULD BE BETTER AT THIS.' WHY SHOULD YOU? YOU ARE STARTING WITH A NEW PROGRAMME, DOING EXERCISES THAT ARE NEW TO YOU, SO NO, YOU SHOULDN'T. NO ONE STARTS OFF DOING THINGS PERFECTLY. WHAT WOULD BE THE FUN IN THAT? WHERE WOULD THE CHALLENGE LIE? ENJOY THE PROCESS AND PROGRESS. ENJOY GETTING BETTER WITH EVERY WEEK. STOP WITH THE 'SHOULDA' BULLSHIT.

WEEKS 1 & 2
PROGRAMME 2 GROUP 2
THREE EXERCISES IN A ROW. FOUR SETS OF EACH.
45-SECOND REST BETWEEN SETS.

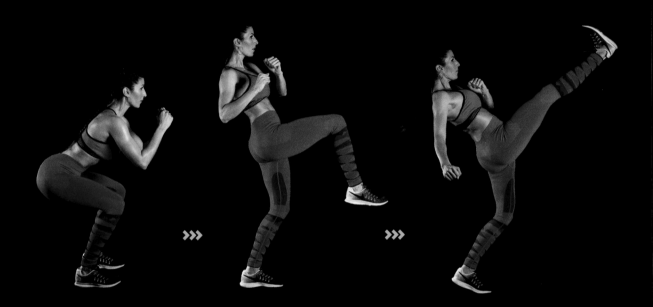

1 SQUAT FORWARD KICK
45 SECONDS ON EACH LEG

>>> Start in your Energy Squat position (see page 41).

>>> Then, at the same time as you come slightly out of that deep powerful position, kick one leg forward as high and with as much power as you can. Think massive power and strength coming out through your heel and smashing someone. In the face. Then land back in the squat and go again! Fast and hard! As you come down, watch that your knees don't bend inwards.

>>> Every time you kick, lean your torso slightly backwards. That way, not only will you kick higher and engage the back muscles of your supporting leg more but you can also go deeper into your core engagement, as you will need to stabilize and balance yourself. Use your arms to generate more power as well. Start with your arms up in front of your head and, as you kick, bring your arms diagonally down on the same side as the kicking leg – like you are bringing an axe down and chopping wood.

>>> Keep on going for 45 seconds, then change legs and repeat for 45 seconds.

2 CRAWLS 30 SECONDS

▶▶▶ Come down into your Root Power High Plank position (see page 41).

▶▶▶ Begin to crawl forward by moving your opposite arm to leg as you move. You should bend your arms and knees as you crawl but not much, and your steps should be short, as you want to keep that plank-straight line of the body – do not let your bum start to lift up.

▶▶▶ Keep moving forward in short fast steps: 6 steps forward, before reversing 6 steps backward. Think Spiderman!

VIKING MENTAL POINTER

WHEN PEOPLE ASK: 'WHAT DO YOU DO?' ANSWER: 'WHATEVER IT TAKES.'

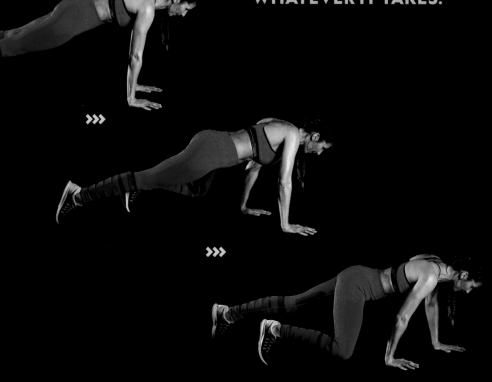

3 PLANK FORWARD REACHES
30 SECONDS

>>> Use a mat for this one. Start in a plank position (see page 41) on your forearms with your shoulders straight above the elbows and hands out in front. Your legs should be hip width apart. Tuck your pelvis under and engage your core. It should be on fire!

>>> Slowly reach one arm forward, lengthening it out so you end with it in a straight line from your shoulder to your fingertips without shifting your body weight. Keep your hips level and still. If you feel your body weight shifting between your feet as you alternate lifting your arms forwards, it means that you are moving your hips too much and losing your core engagement. Engage!

>>> Bring your arm back to that starting position and bring the other arm out.

>>> This is a slow exercise – take your time and maintain control. If you speed it up, you will start shifting your weight and swinging your body, which completely misses the point, which is making your core more powerful. Focus on doing it right.

REMEMBER YOUR POST COOL-DOWN STRETCHES ON PAGES 84–7.

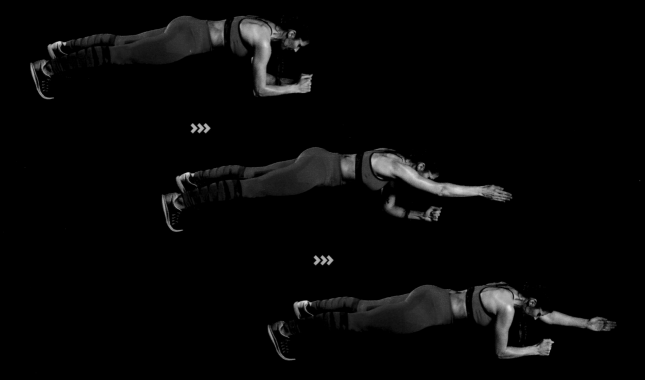

THE VIKING MADNESS

FOUR EXERCISES IN A ROW. FIVE SETS.

ONLY TAKE A BREATHER WHEN YOU NEED TO AND ONLY FOR AS LONG AS YOU ABSOLUTELY NEED TO! WARM UP, GET THAT TIMER READY AND DO NOT STOP UNTIL YOU ARE FINISHED WITH THOSE FIVE SETS. WE DO WHAT WE SET OUT TO DO.

VIKING MENTAL POINTER

IT IS GREAT TO FAIL. FAILURE BREEDS
SUCCESS. EVERY TIME YOU FAIL,
YOU ARE GETTING BETTER. SO NEVER
GIVE UP, BUT KEEP ON FAILING.
KEEP ON PUSHING YOURSELF,
GROWING, EXPANDING.
YOUR TIME NOW, VIKING.

1 SKIPPING 90 SECONDS

>>> Using a skipping rope, skip as fast as you possibly can.

>>> No jump between, keep your core engaged and do small quick jumps.

>>> Keep count! Then every round the aim is to get just a few more reps in!

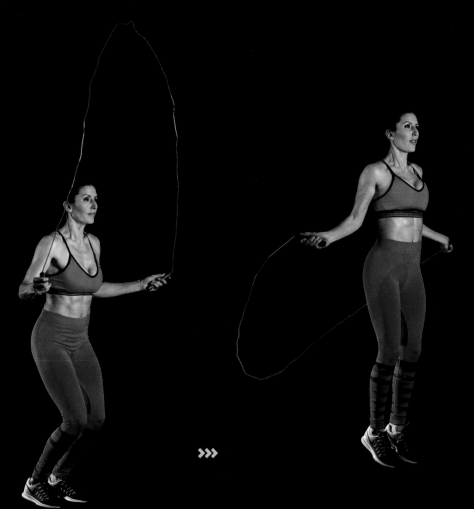

>>>

2 STRAIGHT FORWARD RAISE
14 REPS

>>> Stand, feet facing forward, with your legs a little bit wider than hip width apart. Engage your core, keep your back straight and your shoulders rolled back.

>>> Hold a dumbbell in each hand, with your palms facing each other.

>>> Squat deeply with the weights sinking straight down between your legs. Push your bum back, keeping the weight in your heels and making sure your knees don't come over your toes. Also watch that your shoulders and chest don't roll forward – keep your head up and your eyes on the horizon.

>>> Keep the arms straight as you lift them out in front of you and all the way over your head, straightening the legs at the same time. Keep your core engaged, especially as you bring the weights over your head, as there is a danger of arching your lower back.

>>> Repeat 14 times.

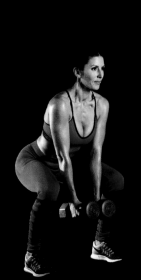 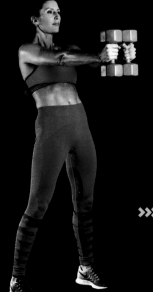 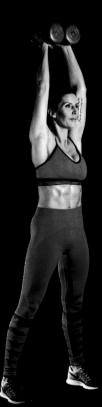

3 DUMBBELL MOVE IN A PLANK
12 SLOW AND CONTROLLED REPS

>>> Use a mat for this one. Start in a plank position (see page 41) on your forearms with your shoulders straight above the elbows and hands out in front. Your legs should be hip width apart. Tuck your pelvis under and engage your core. You should feel the burn!

>>> Place a dumbbell behind the left elbow.

>>> Lift the right hand up without swinging your right hip up (it stays down!) or shifting your weight. Take the weight and move it to the side.

>>> Place the hand back down – the weight should now be behind your right elbow. Repeat with the left hand.

>>> This is proper core work, so be very conscious of doing it technically right, and not arching your lower back or twisting your body. The way you are working your core here is by using it to keep you still. As you lift your arm and move that weight sideways, the core needs to work extra hard to keep the rest of your body still. As soon as you lift the hip on the same side as your working arm and twist it, you lose your core engagement. Keep that hip down by locking it in with your core!

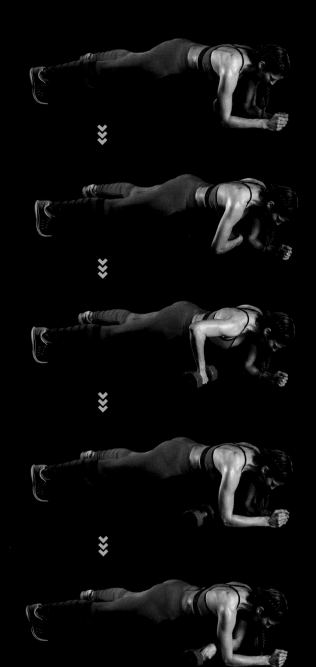

4 SIDE SQUAT JUMP WITH HALF A BURPEE 14 REPS

>>> Place a dumbbell or a rolled-up mat on the floor as a marker.

>>> Stand to the left-hand side of the marker with your feet facing forward and hip width apart. Lower down into a squat, then side jump over the marker and land on the other side still in a squat.

>>> Still in the squat, place your hands on the ground between your legs and jump back with both legs into the Root Power High Plank position (see page 41), engaging your core like mad, then quickly jump back forward into the squat with your heels down and chest up. That is one rep.

Tip: A common mistake is to drop your hips down to the floor and arch your lower back as you jump backwards into that High Plank position. To avoid this, as soon as your feet hit the ground, you need to engage your core like crazy to work against gravity.

REMEMBER YOUR POST COOL-DOWN STRETCHES ON PAGES 84–7.

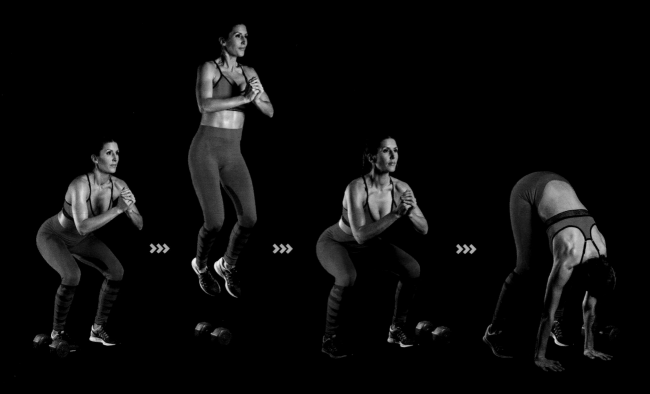

IN THE SECOND TWO WEEKS OF THE PROGRAMME,
YOU SHOULD BE STEPPING ALL OF THIS UP A LEVEL,
DECREASING THE TIME IT TAKES YOU TO DO
THE MADNESS, PUSHING YOURSELF IN ALL THE
PROGRAMMES, GOING DEEPER, FASTER AND
WITH MORE POWER IN ALL THE EXERCISES.
ENJOY WITNESSING YOUR FITNESS AND YOUR
MENTAL RESILIENCE INCREASING.
IT'S ALL DOWN TO YOU AND YOUR HARD WORK.

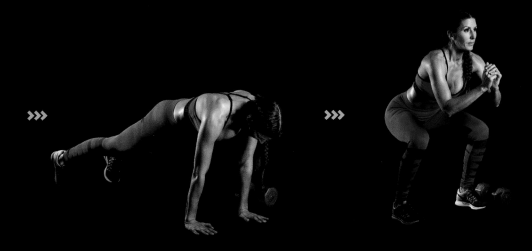

WEEKS 3 & 4
PROGRAMME 3

AFTER YOU HAVE FINISHED ALL THE SETS OF GROUP 1, TAKE A 2-MINUTE REST BEFORE MOVING ON TO GROUP 2 – THIS IS TO CATCH YOUR BREATH AND GET READY FOR THE NEW EXERCISES.

GROUP 1

EXERCISES 1, 2, 3 IN A ROW.

FOUR SETS.

45-SECOND REST BETWEEN SETS.

2-MINUTE REST

GROUP 2

EXERCISES 4, 5, 6 IN A ROW.

FOUR SETS.

45-SECOND REST BETWEEN SETS.

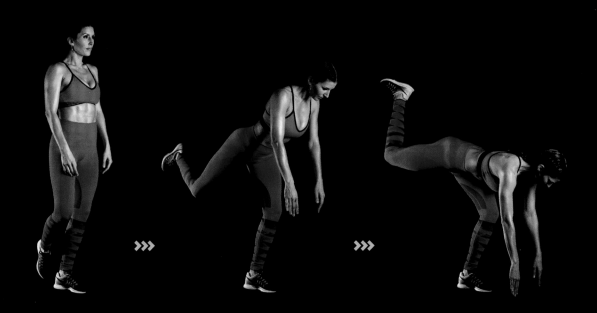

1 ONE-LEGGED SQUAT
30 SECONDS ON EACH LEG

>>> Start in your Battle Stance (see page 40), with your right leg slightly bent backwards and off the floor. Lift the right leg backwards and up, bringing your upper body forwards and downwards and at the same time bend your supporting leg, coming down into a one-legged squat and touching the ground with your hands without putting any weight down on the floor. (Watch that your shoulders stay back and your back remains straight.) Squat as deeply as you can while staying focused and in control.

>>> Extend yourself back out of that squat by going up exactly as you came down in reverse. Stability is hugely helped by the core. So use your core. Engage it, Viking!

>>> Keep on going for 30 seconds, then repeat on the left leg.

Tip: To keep the supporting leg rooted and your body weight going forwards, watch that you bend your supporting leg and keep your body weight back through that backwards bum line.

VIKING MENTAL POINTER

YOU HAVE TO DO BURPEES FOR 45 SECONDS AND THAT IS WORK. BUT WHETHER YOU ARE DOING THINGS THAT ARE GOOD FOR YOUR BODY OR BAD FOR YOUR BODY, BOTH REQUIRE WORK. WHETHER YOU ARE BUILDING YOURSELF UP OR TEARING YOURSELF DOWN MENTALLY, BOTH REQUIRE WORK. AND WHETHER YOU ARE USING YOUR TIME TO GET THE LIFE YOU WANT OR WASTING YOUR TIME IN A LIFE YOU DON'T WANT, BOTH REQUIRE WORK. DON'T FOOL YOURSELF. IT IS ALL WORK. YOU HAVE A CHOICE. YOU CAN EITHER WORK FOR SOMETHING AND REAP THE POSITIVE BENEFITS, OR YOU CAN WORK FOR NOTHING AND EXPERIENCE THE NEGATIVE EFFECTS. MAKE THE WORK WORK FOR YOU. GET READY FOR THOSE 45 SECONDS!

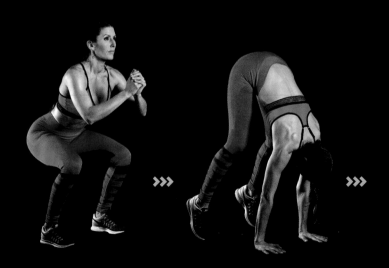

2 BURPEES 45 SECONDS

▶▶▶ Start in your Energy Squat position (see page 41).

▶▶▶ Hands down to the floor between your legs, jump feet backwards into the Root Power High Plank position (see page 41), locking your core in.

▶▶▶ Jump back to the squat, and as you do so, your heels have to be placed down on the ground. This is very important, as when your feet are down, your weight is back and you can truly engage your muscles and work them properly (and you don't put extra pressure on your knees).

▶▶▶ From the squat, jump straight up, bring your arms above your head and land back in the same deep, Energy Squat position. That is one burpee – now how many more can you do in 45 seconds?

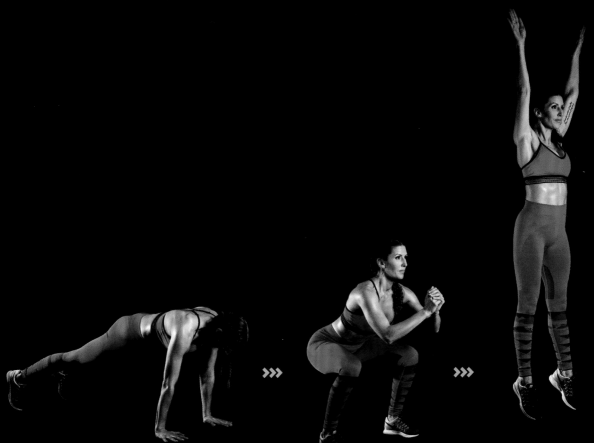

3 WALKING PRESS-UPS 45 SECONDS

⟫⟫ Start in your Battle Stance (see page 40).

⟫⟫ Squat down and bring your hands to the floor, with your back straight, and walk your hands forward until you are in the Root Power High Plank position (see page 41) with your arms slightly wider apart.

⟫⟫ Do a press-up (lower your chest towards the floor then push back up, keeping your body in one straight line and making sure your stomach doesn't sag down – your core and chest should come up at the same time). You can come down on to your knees if you need to, but make sure you keep your body in a straight line from the top of your head right down to your knees. As you come down your elbows should be bending slightly backwards, not flaring straight out to the side.

⟫⟫ Walk your hands back towards your feet, plant your heels down firmly and extend all the way up. Then fold straight back down, no pauses.

Tip: Watch out not to extend your head forwards down to the floor further than your body when you are doing the press-up. Relax your head: it shouldn't be doing any work.

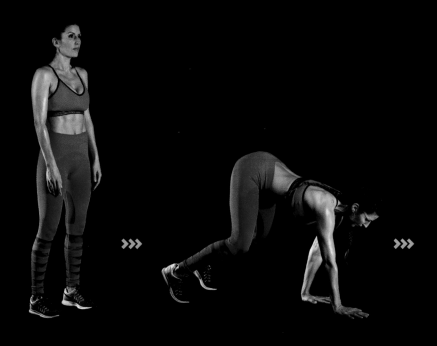

VIKING MENTAL POINTER

CHANGE IS ALWAYS FORCED. IT IS NEVER GIVEN.
NO ONE WILL MAKE IT HAPPEN FOR YOU. FOR THIS,
YOU HAVE TO PULL UP YOUR SOCKS AND DO IT YOURSELF.
YOU HAVE TO RISK IT. YOU HAVE TO GIVE IT YOUR ALL.
YOU HAVE TO GO FOR THINGS IN ORDER TO GET THEM.
YOU CANNOT LET THE FEAR OF FAILING, OF LOSING,
OF LOOKING STUPID, HOLD POWER OVER YOU OR IT
WILL ALWAYS RESULT IN EXACTLY WHAT YOU DIDN'T
WANT. YOU LOSING. YOU MISSING OUT.
GET OFF THE SIDELINES. GET INTO THE GAME.
IT'S YOUR TIME NOW, VIKING.

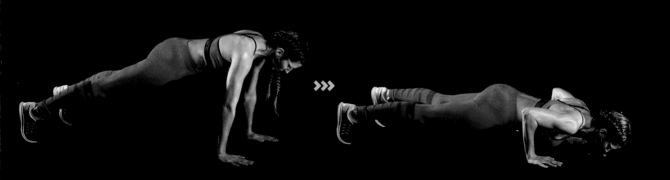

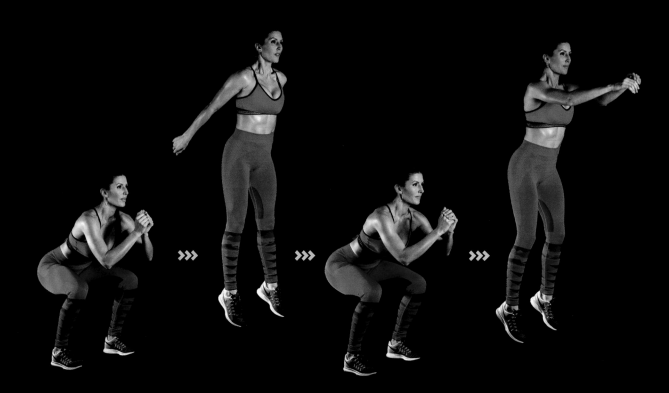

1 FORWARD AND BACKWARD
SQUAT JUMPS 45 SECONDS

>>> Start in your Energy Squat (see page 41).

>>> Jump forward, jump backward. Watch that you always take off and land in a deep squat with your heels down, chest up and shoulders back: don't come up out of the squat after landing, maintain it throughout. And keep up the distance! Jump as far forwards AND as far backwards as you can. Go as deep as you can: the deeper you go, the more you'll feel this exercise. Quick and powerful!

2 ARM WALKS
4 FORWARD, 4 BACKWARD ON TOWELS FOR 30 SECONDS

>>> Stand with each foot on a folded tea towel or magazine and come down into your Root Power High Plank position (see page 41).

>>> Using only your upper body and core, drag your body forward with your hands: four arm steps and then four arm steps backwards. Watch that you don't drop your hips down or arch your back. Engage the core, keep the plank line throughout the exercise, and don't swing your body from side to side! Your hips stay still, squeezing that core to prevent any swinging movement of the body.

Tip: Taking too large arm steps makes it impossible to keep the hips still, while also placing too much pressure on your shoulders. Keep those steps super short!

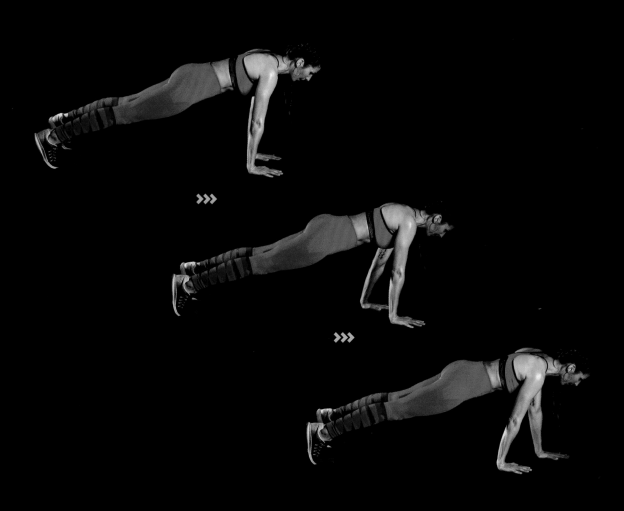

3 **TRICEP KICKBACKS IN A PLANK**
30 SECONDS EACH SIDE

⟩⟩⟩ Use a mat for this one and have a dumbbell to hand. Start in a plank position (see page 57) on your forearms with your shoulders straight above the elbows, and your hands out in front. Your legs should be hip width apart. Tuck your pelvis under and engage your core. If you can't feel it burn, it's not engaged!

⟩⟩⟩ Hold a dumbbell in one hand. Lift the arm holding the dumbbell backwards, keeping it parallel to your body with the elbow bent. Keep the top half of your arm still and lengthen out the lower forearm, working your triceps, then bend the lower part of your arm back in again.

⟩⟩⟩ While you're lifting your arm, focus on making sure the hip on the same side doesn't lift up and twist – it needs to face the floor the whole time. What will keep it down is your core engagement: fire it up!

⟩⟩⟩ Repeat for 30 seconds, then swap arms and do the same on the other side. This exercise should be slow and controlled. You need to stay focused, as you have a lot to think about: keeping your hip down, powering the position through your core, and working the back of your arm by keeping everything else still and contracted while extending the lower arm.

REMEMBER YOUR POST COOL-DOWN STRETCHES ON PAGES 84–7.

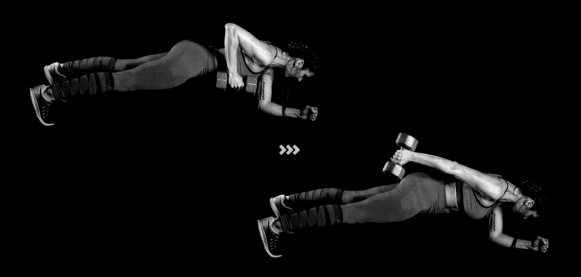

VIKING MENTAL POINTER

IF YOU ARE TRAINING IN FRONT OF A MIRROR, REMEMBER THAT IT IS THERE TO HELP YOU. IT IS THERE FOR YOU TO CHECK YOUR TECHNIQUE AND POSTURE. IT IS THERE FOR YOU TO SEE WHERE TO SWIPE SWEAT OFF. IT IS THERE FOR YOUR BADASS VIKING SELF YOU-GOT-THIS GAME TALK. WHAT IS IT NOT THERE FOR? IT IS NOT THERE FOR YOU TO BELITTLE YOURSELF BY FINDING FAULTS IN THE WAY YOU LOOK. IT IS NOT THERE FOR YOU TO DECREASE YOUR MENTAL ENERGY BY TALKING SHIT ABOUT HOW BAD YOU ARE, HOW AWFUL YOU LOOK IN GYM CLOTHES. STOP USING IT FOR THESE SELF-DESTRUCTIVE THINGS. THEY DO NOT SERVE YOU. FROM NOW ON, USE IT ONLY FOR YOU: TO CHECK YOUR TECHNIQUE, TO WIPE THAT SWEAT AND TO GIVE YOURSELF A FIST PUMP FOR BEING A HARDCORE VIKING. BOOM!

WEEKS 3 & 4
PROGRAMME 4

AFTER YOU HAVE FINISHED ALL THE SETS OF GROUP 1, TAKE A 2-MINUTE REST BEFORE MOVING ON TO GROUP 2 – THIS IS TO CATCH YOUR BREATH AND GET READY FOR THE NEW EXERCISES.

GROUP 1

EXERCISES 1, 2, 3 IN A ROW.

FOUR SETS.

45-SECOND REST BETWEEN SETS.

2-MINUTE REST

GROUP 2

EXERCISES 4, 5, 6 IN A ROW.

FOUR SETS.

45-SECOND REST BETWEEN SETS.

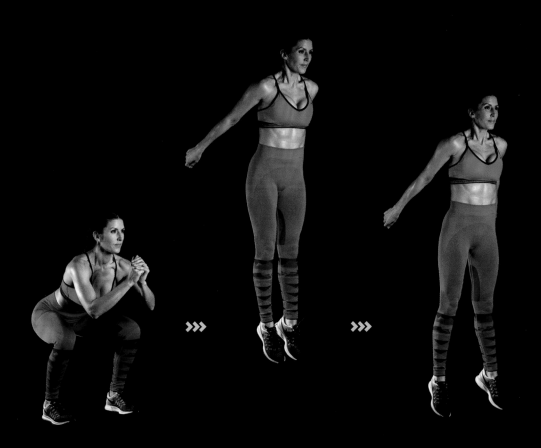

1 NARROW BEATS 30 SECONDS

>>> Come down into your Energy Squat position, full of power and strength (see page 41).

>>> Spring up and, as you jump up, lengthen the legs fully and bring them together in the air with a gentle tap of the inside of your thighs.

>>> Land back straight into that deep squat and repeat for 30 seconds.

Tip: Do straighten your legs fully in the jump – imagine that they are like scissor blades. In the air, close the scissors.

2 KNEELING KICKS 45 SECONDS EACH LEG

⟫ Use a mat for this exercise. Step your left leg far forward and bend the back leg so that you end up in a deep lunge, with your left leg bent at a 90° angle and your right leg bent down with the knee at a 90° angle as well. Keep your torso straight. Now lower that right knee down to the floor, resting the whole of the lower leg on the floor without putting any weight on your toes; your foot should be resting on its instep on the floor. This is your starting position.

⟫ Place your weight through the heel of your front leg and use your hamstrings (the muscles at the back of your upper leg) and the glutes (your bum muscles) of that leg to push up and kick the back leg forward and up. As you kick, lean your torso slightly backward. This way you will be able to kick higher, engage the back muscles of your supporting leg more fully and go deeper

into your core engagement, as you will need to stabilize and balance yourself. Imagine you are kicking someone very tall and slightly out of reach in the face! Thinking that will make you reach your leg forward and lean your torso backward.

⟫ Slowly come back down to that starting position, not letting the lower leg and knee of your back leg touch the floor until you are all the way down – use the muscles in your front leg to control your descent. Repeat for 45 seconds on each leg.

Tip: Don't lean your torso too far forward in order to come up. Yes, you will lean forward a tiny bit, but focus on going straight up. It can also be tempting to use the toes of your back leg to help you come up: don't do it, Viking!

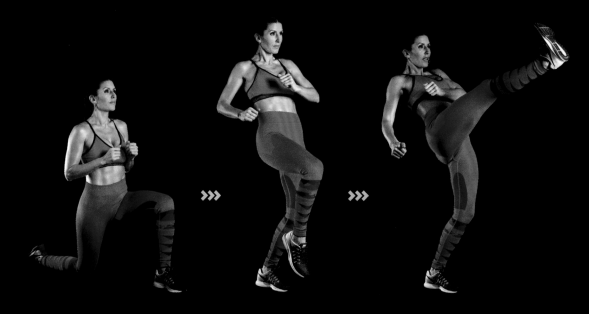

3 **LATERAL RAISES** 30 SECONDS

⋙ Take two dumbbells – if you have more than one set of dumbbells, then try to go for a heavier weight than you have gone for before. We are constantly pushing ourselves!

⋙ Stand in in your Battle Stance position (see page 40), with one weight in each hand. Your shoulders should be back, and your core engaged.

⋙ Lift your arms up sideways, no higher than your shoulders, and back down. Your wrists should not be leading the movement. Imagine that you have a piece of string attached to your deltoid (shoulder muscle)

and that's what's lifting your arms up. It's your shoulders that should be doing the work. Keep your elbows soft, making sure not to lock them.

⋙ Repeat for 30 seconds.

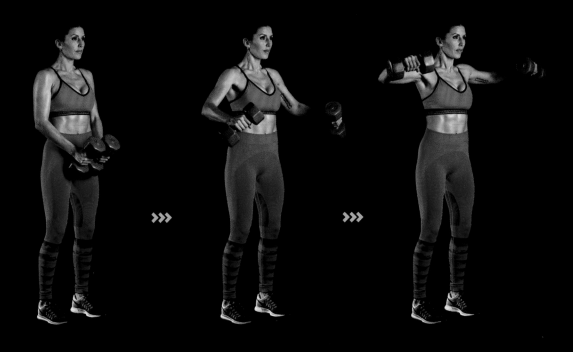

WEEKS 3 & 4
PROGRAMME 4 GROUP 2
THREE EXERCISES IN A ROW. FOUR SETS OF EACH.
45-SECOND REST BETWEEN SETS.

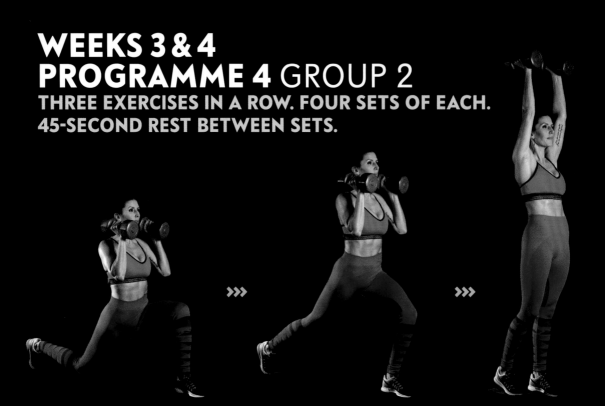

1 BACKWARD SLIDING LUNGE WITH SHOULDER PRESS 45 SECONDS ON EACH LEG

>>> Take two dumbbells, one in each hand, and keep your feet hip width apart. Place a folded tea towel under one foot.

>>> Hold the dumbbells at shoulder level with your elbows tucked in.

>>> Slide the leg with the tea towel underfoot back, with your weight going backward with the leg, as deep as you can go. Make sure to keep the front knee over the foot, forming a right angle. Your back leg should be slightly bent to enable you to go further down and keep your core engaged. Keep your torso upright – no leaning forward.

>>> Engage the back and glutes (bum muscles) of the forward leg, as well as

your core, and use them to drag that leg back in and bring yourself back up to standing.

>>> At the same time, as you are coming up, press your arms upward with your palms facing each other, to a full straight arm shoulder press.

>>> Lower yourself back down into that deep backward sliding lunge and bring your hands back to shoulder level as you reach the bottom of your lunge. Make sure your front knee isn't overshooting when you come back down. Repeat for 45 seconds on each leg. This is a continuous compound movement, therefore do not break it up. As your leg goes backward, your weights go down; as your leg comes back forward, your weights go up.

2 PLANK SHIFTER 30 SECONDS

>>> Come down to your Root Power High Plank position (see page 41).

>>> From there, without swinging or twisting your hips, place your left forearm down on the floor followed by your right forearm, bringing yourself down into the plank on forearms position. Then, slowly and with as much control as possible from your core, come back up on to your left palm and then your right, bringing yourself back into that starting position. Keep your body as still as you can and, as you come up, put the palm underneath your body (it should sit under your upper chest) so you feel the movement more in your core rather than just in your shoulders. Do not swing your hips!

>>> Alternate which forearm you go down on first. Continue for 30 seconds.

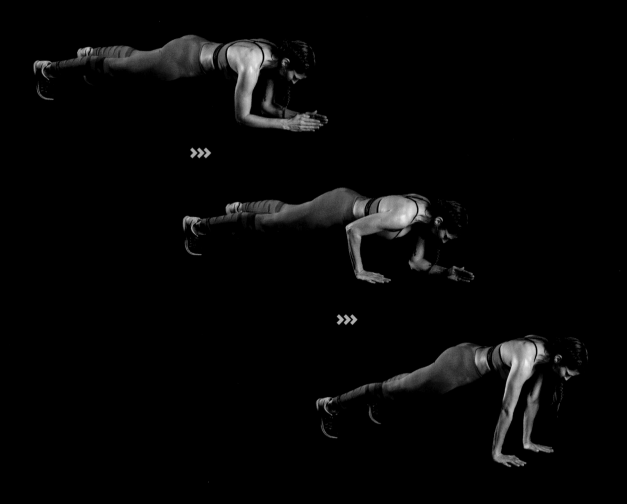

3 **VIKING LAY DOWNS** 45 SECONDS

⟫⟫ Start in your Battle Stance (see page 40) with tea towels under each foot. Bring your hands down to the floor, with your arms straight, and legs slightly bent.

⟫⟫ Then slide the legs back, and as soon as your body is in a parallel line to the floor, bring yourself all the way down to the floor. Your arms should be bending upwards with the elbows tucked in.

⟫⟫ Really fire up your core, as that engagement is what will fuel you to come back up. Lift your body up off the floor in a straight line, slide your legs in, keep your bum up, and end up in a folded position

with your knees slightly bent. Then release your arms off the floor and extend your torso up, ending back in that strong Battle Stance position.

⟫⟫ Repeat for 45 seconds.

Tip: Don't forget about your core! Even though this exercise involves resting your body on the floor, your core should always be working, keeping everything in place and driving the movement.

Tip: As always, you can switch the tea towels for magazines if you are slaying the programme on a carpet.

REMEMBER YOUR POST COOL-DOWN STRETCHES ON PAGES 84–7.

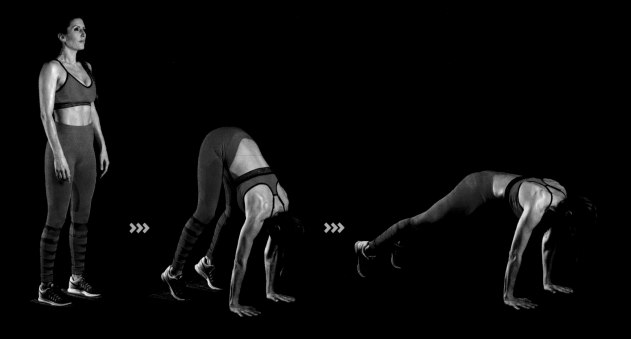

VIKING MENTAL POINTER

WITH EACH EXERCISE THAT YOU ARE DOING,
ESPECIALLY THE MORE CHALLENGING ONES,
I WANT YOU TO ONLY THINK ABOUT THAT EXERCISE.
NOT ABOUT ALL THE OTHER ONES THAT YOU HAVE LEFT
TO DO. THIS CAN MAKE IT OVERWHELMING AND MORE
DIFFICULT MENTALLY TO FINISH THE PROGRAMME.
THEREFORE, ONLY THINK ABOUT FINISHING
THIS EXERCISE. JUST GET TO THE END OF THIS ONE.
THERE IS ONLY YOU AND THIS EXERCISE.

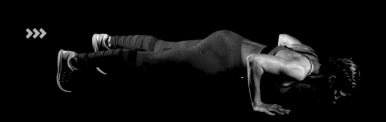

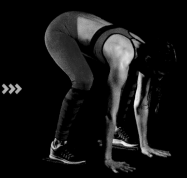

THE VIKING MADNESS

FOUR EXERCISES IN A ROW.
FIVE SETS.
SLAY, VIKING, SLAY!

THE MADNESS IN WEEKS 3 & 4 IS THE SAME AS IN WEEKS 1 & 2 (TURN TO PAGES 58–63).

VIKING MENTAL POINTER

IF YOU WANT THINGS TO CHANGE, THEN YOU HAVE
TO CHANGE. IF YOU WANT MORE, THEN YOU HAVE
TO BECOME MORE. IF YOU WANT THINGS TO IMPROVE,
THEN YOU HAVE TO IMPROVE. THAT IS WHAT YOU
ARE DOING RIGHT NOW. YOU ARE MAGNIFYING YOUR
SKILLS INSTEAD OF MODIFYING YOUR DREAMS.
GIVE YOURSELF A HUGE WELL DONE FOR THAT.
AND NOW WE WILL KEEP ON GOING!

THE VIKING MADNESS

1 SKIPPING
90 SECONDS

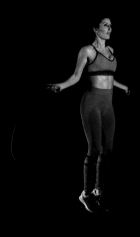

2 STRAIGHT FORWARD RAISE
14 REPS

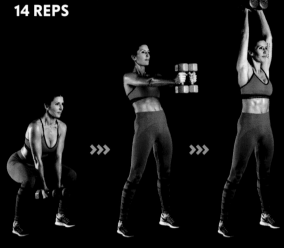

3 DUMBBELL MOVE IN A PLANK
12 SLOW & CONTROLLED REPS

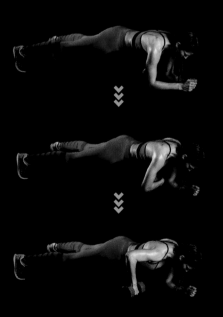

4 SIDE SQUAT JUMP WITH HALF A BURPEE
14 REPS

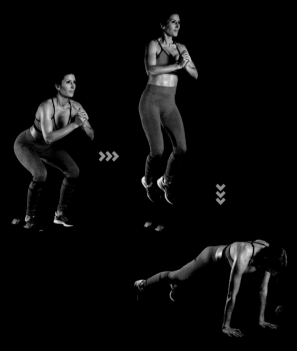
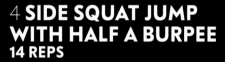

POST COOL-DOWN STRETCHES

DO ALL THESE STRETCHES IN A ROW AFTER YOU FINISH YOUR PROGRAMME AND YOUR COOL-DOWN.

#1

Lie on your back. Keep your right leg down on the floor, lift the left leg up and grab the back of it with your hands. Pull the leg gently towards your head, keeping your hips down. Keep your neck relaxed. Don't pulse the leg (move it in and out of the stretch in a pulsing manner). Breathe in, and every time you breathe out pull your leg a little bit closer to you. Hold the stretch for 30–60 seconds on each leg.

#2

Lie on your back. Bend your right leg with your knee facing up to the sky. Lift your left leg and turn it out, bending it down so that your knee faces out to the side, and place the side of your foot just above the knee of your right leg. Feed your hands through, grab behind the thigh of your right leg and pull it towards your head. Keep your neck and shoulders relaxed. Hold the stretch for 30–60 seconds on each leg.

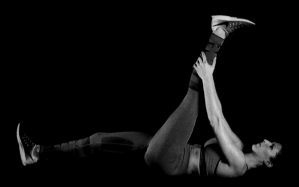

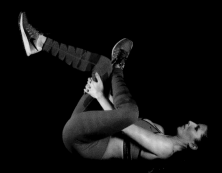

#3

Sit upright with your legs straight in front of you. Lift through your spine, lengthening and straightening up your torso. Take the left arm and place it on the outside of the right leg. Keep it straight. Press the arm against the leg and twist your torso to the right. Your right arm reaches backwards and you are looking along that right arm. Use the pressing of the arm against the leg to constantly go further into that backwards twist. Hold for 30–60 seconds on each side.

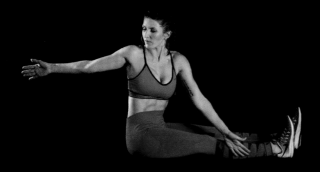

#4

Come into a Downward Dog position: Start on all fours. Tuck your toes under and lift your knees off the floor. Press into the palms of your hands, stretch your elbows, relax your upper back. Reach your bum up to the sky, gently lengthening your legs. Straighten your knees but do not lock them. Press your heels down to the floor, bringing your body into the shape of an A. Extend your knees, lift your bum up, and keep your back straight, with your head in between your arms. Align your ears with your upper arms. Relax your neck. Press your chest towards your thighs, feeling the lengthening of your spine, and at the same time press your heels further down to the floor, feeling the lengthening of the backs of your legs. Hold for 30–60 seconds. Then put all your weight on your left leg, swing the right leg up, keeping it straight, bend it and open your right hip outwards, making the lower right leg drop to the outside of the left leg line. This will open up your hip flexor and stretch your quads. Hold for 30–60 seconds on each leg.

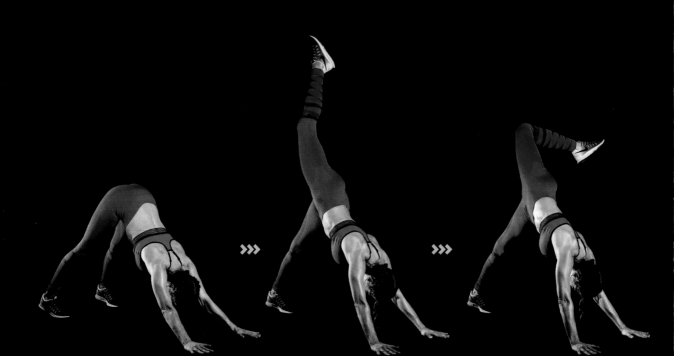

#5

Stand up straight, breathe in and lengthen up through your spine. Lift your right hand up, and lean your body to the left with the arm stretching over your head. Feel your right side stretch. At the same time, to feel the stretch deeper, press down into your right heel, placing force down through your right leg to the floor, which will make it a proper two-way stretch; the right side of your upper body stretching upward and over to the side and your right leg lengthening down into the floor. After you have done both sides for 30–60 seconds each, lift both arms up, opening them slightly, look up, broadening your chest, and press your arms slightly backward. Breathe deeply in and out and enjoy feeling long, stretched and powerful after smashing your workout.

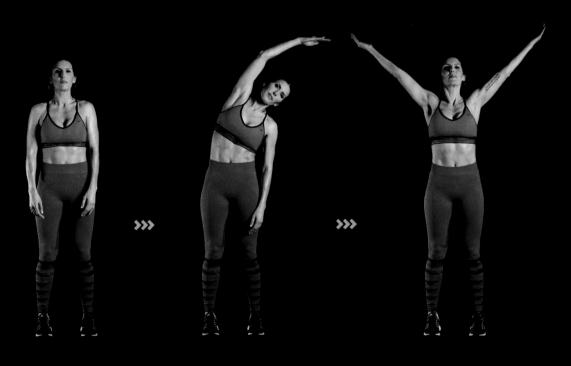

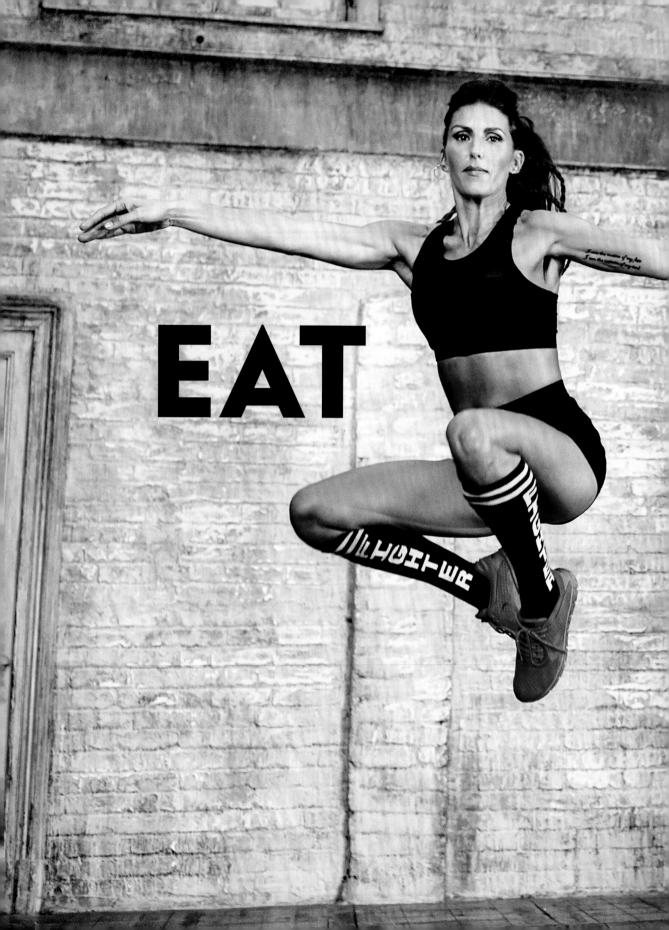

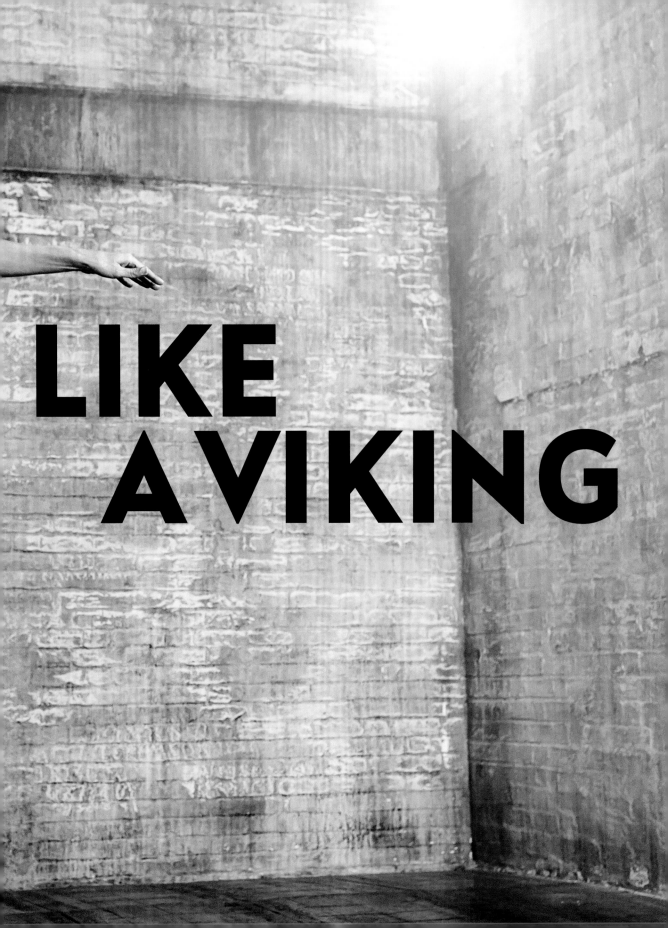

» VIKINGS EAT A BALANCED DIET

Nutrition is all about bringing your body into balance: full of energy, vitality and optimum functioning of all your systems.

» VIKINGS DO NOT COUNT CALORIES

A healthy diet is not about counting each calorie or weighing every single gram of food, but making healthier choices every day.

» VIKINGS ARE IN CONTROL OF THEIR OWN DIET

In the Viking Method, I advise you on what types of food are good to have and suggest guidelines, recipes and meal plans. But I don't break down every single gram of every single meal. That's just not a sustainable way to live. It is horribly boring, time-consuming and antisocial too. The end goal of the weekly meal plan is not to have to use the weekly meal plan. Eating like a Viking is about learning which foods are great to have and, crucially, **when to have them**, and choosing the recipes that suit your taste and lifestyle best, while also being healthy. It's about empowerment rather than restriction.

» VIKINGS ARE ALWAYS READY

Preparation is key. Take food with you to work (check out My Ugly Lunch Box on pages 193–203). Know what you are going to have for dinner. Don't shop when you're hungry, and always make sure you have little snacks on you for when hunger strikes – things you can grab easily, like nuts or an apple, for example. The alternative is a recipe for ending up in the bakery (my weakness – damn you, freshly baked cookies!).

» VIKINGS EAT TO FUEL THEIR TRAINING

On training days you need additional fuel. You are using up more energy that needs replenishing, and in addition you need extra energy to fuel the growth and repair of your muscles. This is why, on training days, you should have a higher amount of carbohydrates to balance against your energy expenditure. Protein and fat are of course also needed. On training days it is also very important to have your carbohydrates at certain times, to get the most out of them and utilize them properly. To make it easier for you, all the Viking recipes are split into Training Days and Anytime recipes that also include advice on when to have your carbs and what carbs to have.

VIKING MANTRA #9
NO MATTER WHAT IS HAPPENING, NO MATTER WHAT OBSTACLES YOU MIGHT FACE, AND NO MATTER HOW DIFFICULT IT MAY SEEM, KNOW THAT YOU CAN SEE IT THROUGH. WHATEVER IT IS, IT IS A TEMPORARY SITUATION. YOU WILL BE OK. YOU ARE STRONG ENOUGH TO FACE IT AND POWERFUL ENOUGH TO FINISH IT. YOU'VE GOT THIS.

MACROS AND MICROS

Nutrients can be split into macronutrients and micronutrients.

Macronutrients = Protein, Fats and Carbs
We need all of these in large amounts, to fuel, repair, grow, maintain and regulate our bodily functions.

Micronutrients = Vitamins and Minerals
We need these in smaller amounts but they are still absolutely essential for healthy growth and development, energy balance, chemical reactions and so on. The well-balanced diet of the Viking Method supplies the micros that you need.

LOW-DOWN ON THE MACROS

PROTEIN

The word 'protein' is derived from the Greek word *protos*, meaning of prime importance. Protein consists of amino acids; and there are 20 amino acids, 9 of which are essential because the body cannot make them itself, they must come from your diet.

Protein is found in every cell in your body. Except for water, protein is the most abundant substance in your body. It is absolutely vital for your body and needs to be constantly replaced. Protein is needed for the maintenance of your body tissue, its development and repair. It is also involved in the creation of some of your hormones, like insulin and secretin.

Enzymes, which are essential for most chemical reactions in the body, are proteins. Protein is a major element in transportation of certain molecules – for example, haemoglobin, which transports oxygen throughout the body, is protein. Protein forms antibodies that help prevent infection, illness and disease.

Good Organic Viking Protein
Animal
» Pastured chicken
» Turkey
» Eggs
» Grass-fed beef
» Wild-caught fish, such as salmon, cod
» Goat's milk feta or sheep's and goat's milk halloumi cheeses (see page 18 for why I choose goat's milk)

Plant
» Seeds, such as sunflower and pumpkin seeds
» A range of legumes: my favourites are kidney beans (NB legumes are high in carbohydrates, therefore if you are not a vegetarian or a vegan, legumes are Sometimes Carbs)
» Nuts, such as cashews and almonds

FATS

Fats do not make you fat.
Fats are absolutely essential for you and their role is much deeper than just as a source of fuel and insulation. Fats help to protect and run your immune system and keep all of your cells working properly. They are needed for the production of Vitamin D as well as of testosterone and oestrogen. Fats are broken down into saturated, unsaturated and trans fats. The good fats are really good; just remember that they are calorific, meaning they pack a lot of energy, therefore watch your intake of them in the normal sense of not overeating.

Unsaturated fats

Unsaturated fats improve blood cholesterol levels, ease inflammation, stabilize heart rhythms and more.

There are two types of good unsaturated fats:

Monounsaturated fats
» Olive oil
» Peanut oil
» Avocado
» Nuts, such as almonds, hazelnuts and pecans
» Seeds, such as pumpkin and sesame

Polyunsaturated fats
» Walnuts
» Flaxseeds
» Flaxseed oil
» Fish
» Rapeseed oil has the lowest saturated fat levels of any oil, and is high in essential fatty acids and a great source of vitamin K and E, which variously strengthen the immune system and help wounds to heal properly. It also has an exceptionally high burning point, which means that heat does not break down its fats nor destroy its flavour and texture, making it excellent for cooking food at high temperatures.
» Omega-3 fats are a very important type of polyunsaturated fat. The body cannot make these itself, therefore they need to come from your diet. A great way to get omega-3 fats is having fish three times a week. For vegetarians and vegans, chia seeds, hemp seeds and walnuts are all good sources of omega-3.

Saturated Fats

Saturated fats are mainly found in animal foods, but are also high in a few plant-based foods.

Good saturated fats
» Beef
» Chicken
» Turkey
» Eggs
» Coconut oil
» Coconut

Trans Fats

These are 'bad fats'; try to eliminate these from your diet. Trans fats are made from heating vegetable oils in the presence of hydrogen gas and a catalyst, a process called hydrogenation. This process converts the oil into solids and makes them withstand repeated heating without breaking down – ideal for frying, baked goods, processed snack foods and margarine.

Trans fats raise the bad cholesterol LDL, which transports cholesterol to your arteries where it can build up and result in a stroke or a heart attack, and lowers the good cholesterol HDL, which transports cholesterol to the liver where it is expelled from the body. Trans fats create inflammation and contribute to insulin resistance (which can lead to type 2 diabetes), and even in small amounts they have harmful health effects that are implicated in heart diseases, stroke and other chronic conditions.

The Viking diet includes the good saturated and unsaturated fats. They are absolutely essential. One of the biggest misconceptions people have is that low-fat products are better for you than full-fat. Generally, when fat – which is full of flavour – has been removed, a huge amount of sugar has been added as a substitute. Avoid anything labelled low-fat.

CARBOHYDRATES

Carbohydrates are made up of sugar molecules, which your body breaks down into fuel. Sugar, carbs and starches are all forms of carbohydrates. There are two main types: simple and complex.

Simple: sweets, cookies, sodas, white rice, white pasta

Complex: brown rice, lentils, apples, quinoa, oats, broccoli

Your body takes both the simple and the complex carbs and breaks them into usable sugars to fuel your muscles and organs. What is important is to understand how quickly the carbs you are having spike up your insulin levels, and to be conscious of when you are eating them.

The complex carbs are slow-releasing carbs, meaning they don't activate that fast insulin spike. But they are still broken down into sugars and if you have too much, that sugar is turned into fat.

The best carbs are the complex fibrous ones. The more fibre they contain, the less impact they have on your hormones. Fibrous complex carbs are vegetables and fruits like broccoli, spinach and avocado (see recipes like the Pesto Chicken & Sweet Potato One-tray Wonder on page 124, the Veggie Hummus Wrap on page 152, and the Icelandic-inspired Poached Cod on page 169), which are packed with the vitamins and minerals that you need, cleanse the liver and are anti-inflammatory. Have loads of vegetables and fibrous fruits throughout the day. They are absolute gold for you and your body.

Vegetable smoothies are also a good everyday option, like my favourite Odin's Green & Mean smoothie (recipe on page 223), as are veggies with your meals. If there is a vegetable that you do not like at all but you know it's good for you, throw it into your smoothie.

Viking carbs mostly come in the form of vegetables and fruits and lots of them – low GI foods which contain slow-releasing carbs that do not spike up insulin levels. You can have these carbs – the Always Carbs – any time. Other complex carbs – the Sometimes Carbs (lentils, rice, oats, quinoa, sweet potatoes) – are only for after you train or for breakfast on your training days.

The Glycemic Index (GI) is a ranking of carbohydrates in foods based on how they affect blood glucose levels. Carbs that are considered low GI have 55 or less, medium have 56—69, and high have 70 or more. Most vegetables have a low GI. Some examples of low GI fruits are: strawberries, pears, apples, plums, kiwi, grapes, oranges.

DRINKS

Vikings drink water and lots of it. Stay hydrated. Drink coffee in moderation (as little as you can) and switch normal tea for herbal. Drink hot water with lemon when you wake up – lemon contains vitamin C and potassium, and having it first thing in the morning gives the body time to absorb the vitamins and minerals properly, plus giving you a little immune system boost.

Drink water throughout the day. Use almond or coconut milk instead of cow's milk. Limit your alcohol intake as much as you can – though Vikings do enjoy a beer every now and then.

SUMMARY OF THE VIKING METHOD OF NUTRITION

» The Always Carbs (see page 11):
  › Eat them any day, at any time, in moderation.
  › Eat a lot of vegetables throughout the day.
  › Only eat fruit that has a low GI, e.g. apples, pears and berries. Fruit that has a high GI should be eaten combined with vegetables, protein or fat, so either within one of your main meals or in a smoothie.

» The Sometimes Carbs (see pages 11 and 224–9):
  › Only to be eaten for breakfast on training days and after you train. Recipes are divided into groups (Training Day and Rest Day Breakfast, Post-training Meals and Anytime Meals), making it easy to know what to eat when.

» If you train before breakfast, you have your Training Day Breakfast (see pages 106–15) straight afterwards and you should also have a Post-training Meal (see pages 118–57) at lunchtime.

» Change your cow's dairy products for goat's, sheep's, almond, soya or coconut dairy-free substitutes.

» Always be prepared. Know what you are going to have for each meal and try to take lunch with you when you're out and about.

» Enjoy food but try not to focus on it. Get your planning done, then forget about it.

» Buy organic wherever possible: fruit and vegetables, as well as tinned beans and pulses.

» Protein (see list of protein-rich foods on page 91) should be eaten at every main meal.

» Only eat GOOD fats, for example, fish, avocado, nuts – always cook with coconut oil or cold-pressed rapeseed oil; olive oil is only for dressing salads.

» Drink LOTS of water, limit your coffee and try to switch to herbal tea.

» Always allow 90 minutes from when you begin eating dinner until you go to sleep, to allow sufficient time for your insulin levels to decrease. The first 90 minutes of sleep have the highest level of growth hormone (fat-burning hormone) and it can only do its job if the insulin levels have gone down.

» Do not eat ANY carbs 90 minutes before exercising. We want your fat-burning hormones to be able to properly kick in. Therefore you might have to move your snacks until after exercising or have them with a meal.

All this is within your control.

You've got this.

THE VIKING DIET

All the recipes that follow are for what I consider to be average-size portions. How much you need to eat depends on several factors, including how active you are during the day. It makes sense that someone who moves around constantly will need more energy than someone who sits at a desk for 8 hours. Eat until you are full but not exploding. You shouldn't feel uncomfortable after eating. If you feel you need more or less, then go by that.

Historically, everything that the Vikings ate was fresh and wild, and although our lifestyle has evolved in many ways, the Viking diet is inspired by that principle where possible. Vegetables. Fruit. Nuts and seeds. Wild-caught fish. Grass-fed meat.

Where possible, buy organic: eggs, tinned beans and pulses, and fresh, organic fruit and vegetables.

Mix and match – there are lots of variations and suggestions given throughout so that you can tailor each recipe to suit you. Everything in here is good for you, so feel free to substitute vegetables, swap chicken for fish and so on. Or follow them to the letter. The aim is to get comfortable with cooking, and to know that what you make doesn't always have to look great (though it will taste it), or be fancy.

Prior to this, if your diet consisted of lots of sweet things and simple sugars, your taste buds and your palate will have become used to that. You will need to 're-train' them into liking less sugary flavours. Therefore, in the beginning, it might take a while to adjust. But think about what all these great nutrients are giving you! Eventually, you will have a very sugary drink, or some cake, and you will find it sickly.

Recipes serve one person, unless otherwise stated.

VIKING MANTRA #10

STAND UP. ROCK THE LONGBOAT. TAKE UP SPACE. BE A HANDFUL. LIVE BY YOUR OWN VALUES AND CONVICTIONS. KEEP YOUR INTEGRITY NO MATTER WHAT OPPORTUNITIES COME YOUR WAY. AND ALWAYS GO TO BED BEING AT PEACE WITH WHO YOU ARE.

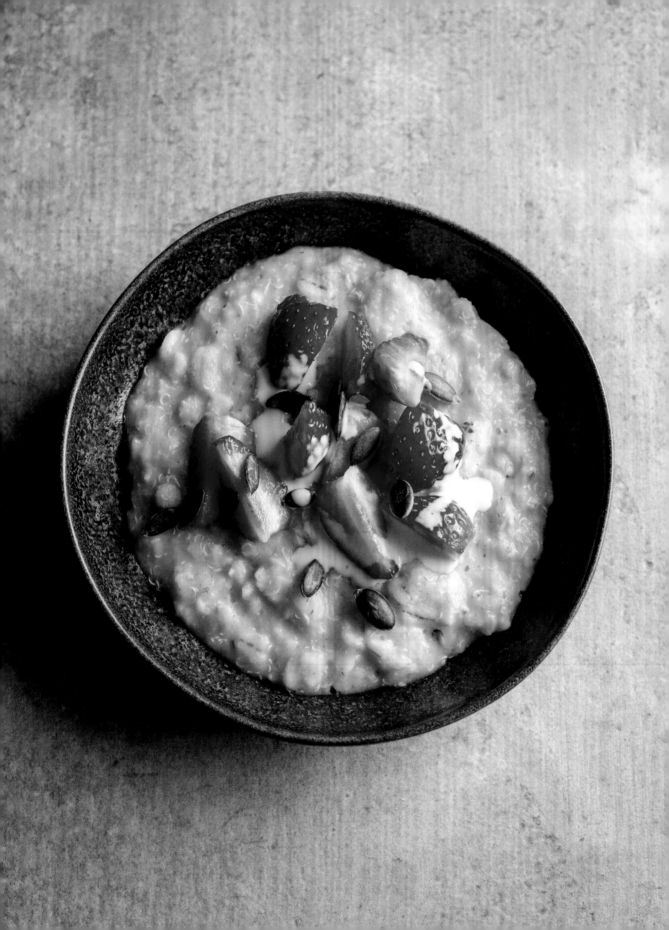

BREAKFAST

On rest days we welcome the day with a breakfast that is high in protein and healthy fats, with our carb intake coming from the Always Carbs, vegetables and fibrous fruits. Training days kick off with slow-releasing, high-fibre carbs, such as oats and chia porridge. Choose from different toppings to keep it interesting. Viking energy is needed for the berserkness of the day!

REST DAY BREAKFASTS

These recipes are all high in quality protein, healthy fats and vitamins and minerals.

In addition, the Viking Smoothies (see Snacks, page 221–3) work really well for breakfast. I start most days with a smoothie and usually add a boiled egg on the side for extra protein and fat, and to keep me fuller for longer. Everyone's needs are different and, if you're a straight-out-the-door type person, you might prefer to have something really simple to fuel you: a couple of boiled eggs and a small handful of almonds, say. Prepare the eggs the night before (see page 119 for instructions on how to boil eggs, if you don't have your own preferred method). Just watch you don't eat on the go – even if it's a small meal, you should always take a few minutes to sit and focus on just eating.

REST DAY BREAKFASTS
SALMON & VEGGIES

Vikings eat loads of fish! It's a different sort of cooked breakfast, but this is a fantastic meal full of hearty, healthy fats that do wonders for you. The perfect way to start the day. Instead of the salmon you could have chicken fillets, but then you'd miss out on those gorgeous omega fats. You don't need to add any oil, as the salmon is steamed, which keeps it nice and juicy.

SERVES 1

1–2 SALMON FILLETS

SEA SALT AND FRESHLY GROUND BLACK PEPPER

A GENEROUS PINCH OF PAPRIKA

½ A RED ONION, THINLY SLICED

3 SPEARS OF ASPARAGUS, ROUGHLY CHOPPED

4–5 BROCCOLI FLORETS, ROUGHLY CHOPPED

1 Preheat the oven to 200°C/180°C fan/gas 6.

2 Line a roasting tray with a piece of tin foil large enough to completely cover the salmon. Place the salmon fillets in the centre and season with salt, pepper and a generous pinch of paprika.

3 Add the red onion, asparagus and broccoli, then fold the foil over to make a parcel (make sure it's properly closed so no steam can escape) and place in the oven.

4 Cook for 20 minutes, then remove from the foil and eat.

AVOCADO WITH SALMON & DILL-LEMON YOGHURT

This delicious breakfast feels luxurious but couldn't be more simple: a meal fit for a Viking on a rest day.

SERVES 1

2 TBSP GOAT'S MILK YOGHURT

25G FRESH DILL, CHOPPED

JUICE OF ½ A LEMON

SEA SALT AND FRESHLY GROUND BLACK PEPPER

1 SMALL AVOCADO

2 SLICES OF SMOKED SALMON

1 TBSP PUMPKIN SEEDS (OPTIONAL)

1 Mix together the yoghurt and dill in a small bowl, and add the lemon juice and salt and pepper to taste.

2 Halve the avocado, remove the stone, and peel off the skin so you're left with two boat-like halves.

3 Fill the hollow in each avocado half with a slice of salmon, and drizzle over the herby dressing. Sprinkle over the pumpkin seeds, if using.

VEGGIE OPTION: Replace the salmon with sweet roasted cherry tomatoes. Cooking tomatoes concentrates their sweet flavour, as well as better enabling us to absorb the antioxidant lycopene. Win, win! Preheat the oven to 180°C/160°C fan/gas 4. Put 8–10 halved cherry tomatoes on a small foil-lined baking tray and drizzle over ½ teaspoon of cold-pressed rapeseed oil. Season with salt and pepper and roast for 15 minutes.

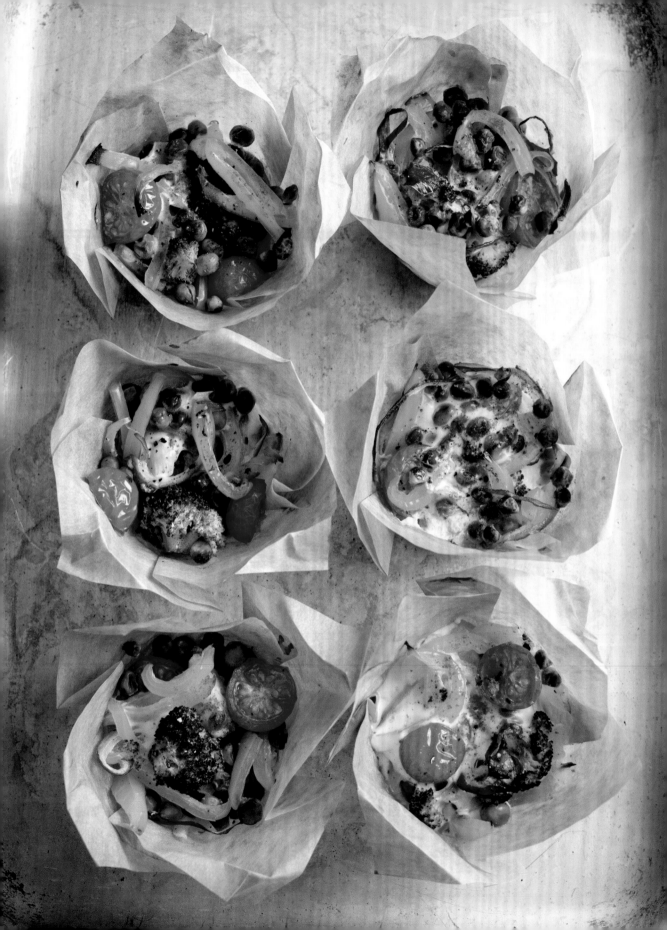

VEGGIE FRITTATAS

These are absolutely brilliant for making ahead, perfect for busy mornings when there's no time to cook.

MAKES 6 MUFFINS, OR 3 PORTIONS

10 SMALL BROCCOLI FLORETS, STEAMED

2 PEPPERS (ANY COLOUR YOU WANT), DESEEDED AND SLICED

1 LARGE TOMATO, CHOPPED, OR 12 CHERRY TOMATOES, HALVED

120G FROZEN PEAS

½ A RED ONION, THINLY SLICED

4 EGGS

SEA SALT AND FRESHLY GROUND BLACK PEPPER

A PINCH OF GROUND CAYENNE PEPPER

1 Preheat the oven to 200°C/180°C fan/gas 6.

2 Mix all the vegetables together in a bowl, and spoon equal amounts into a 6-holed silicone muffin tray (or greaseproof paper cases or a regular muffin tray, greased).

3 Beat the eggs together in a jug, season with salt and pepper and the cayenne, and pour into the muffin holes over the veggies.

4 Bake for about 15–20 minutes, until the eggs are set and cooked through. Leave to cool slightly before removing from the tray.

OPTION: Add greens alongside for an extra nutrient boost: blanch broccoli, asparagus or spinach for a couple of minutes in a pan of boiling water.

OMELETTES: FOUR WAYS

Eggs are among the most nutritious foods you can eat, with whole eggs containing an amazing array and amount of nutrients. Eggs are packed with high-quality protein and fat, vitamins and minerals. The white carries most of the protein and the yolk most of the fat, plus the vitamins and the minerals. In the past, people were warned about eating too many eggs, as they contain cholesterol, but this advice is now out of date. Eggs raise the good cholesterol and change the profile of the bad cholesterol in your body, making it less harmful. What's more, they are exceptionally versatile and, in omelette form, a great vehicle for adding veg to.

JOINT EFFORT

Having healthy joints is crucial. The ingredients in this Viking special are filled with anti-inflammatory, cleansing properties to keep you strong, nimble and in great health.

SERVES 1

2 LARGE EGGS

SEA SALT AND FRESHLY GROUND BLACK PEPPER

COCONUT OR COLD-PRESSED RAPESEED OIL

½ A RED OR YELLOW PEPPER, DESEEDED AND THINLY SLICED

¼ OF AN ONION, THINLY SLICED

1 SMALL TOMATO, CHOPPED

40G KALE, WASHED AND CHOPPED

A SPRIG OF FRESH ROSEMARY, LEAVES PICKED

A PINCH OF GROUND TURMERIC

1 Whisk the eggs in a bowl and season with salt and pepper.

2 Pour a drizzle of oil into a frying pan and place on a medium to high heat. When hot, add the red or yellow pepper and the onion. Cook for a minute, then add the tomato and cook for another minute, stirring. Finally add the kale and cook for 1 more minute, then remove everything in the pan to a plate.

3 Wipe the pan with a piece of kitchen paper if necessary, then add a little more oil and return the pan to the heat. Pour in the eggs and cook on a high heat for 2 minutes, making sure that the egg mixture is spread out evenly.

4 As the eggs begin to set, lower the heat and add the veg mixture to one half of the pan, sprinkling over the rosemary leaves and turmeric.

5 Use a spatula to free the edges, then fold the omelette over and serve.

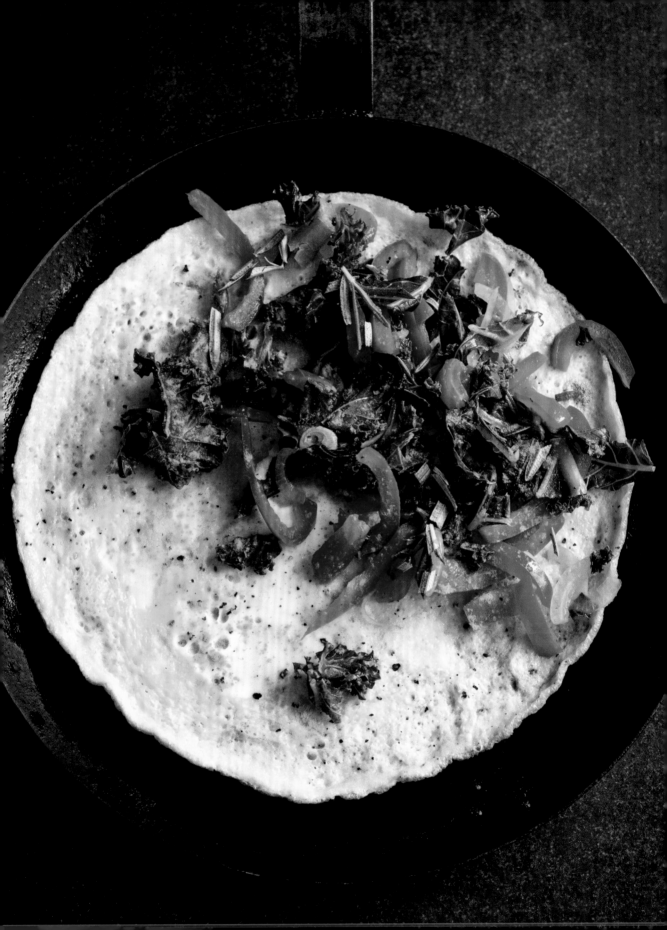

IMMUNITY

Cherry tomatoes are one of the richest sources of vitamin C, which you need to keep your immune system in tip-top shape, and garlic contains a compound, allicin, that helps your immune system fight germs. You're ready for anything, Viking!

SERVES 1

2 LARGE EGGS

SEA SALT AND FRESHLY GROUND BLACK PEPPER

COCONUT OR COLD-PRESSED RAPESEED OIL

3 CHERRY TOMATOES, HALVED

½ A CLOVE OF GARLIC, CHOPPED

3 WHITE MUSHROOMS, SLICED

1 Whisk the eggs in a bowl and season with salt and pepper.

2 Pour a drizzle of oil into a frying pan and place on a medium to high heat. When hot, add the tomatoes, garlic and mushrooms. Cook, stirring, until the veggies soften and start to colour, then remove to a plate and return the pan to the heat.

3 Add a little more oil to the pan, then pour in the eggs. Cook on a high heat for 2 minutes, making sure that the egg mixture is spread out evenly.

4 As the eggs begin to set, lower the heat and add the veggies to one half of the pan.

5 Use a spatula to free the edges, then fold the omelette over and serve.

TAKE OFF!

The ingredients in this energy-boosting omelette will lift you into high slaying mode, making you ready for anything that comes your way!

SERVES 1

2 LARGE EGGS

SEA SALT AND FRESHLY GROUND BLACK PEPPER

COCONUT OR COLD-PRESSED RAPESEED OIL

2 COOKED TURKEY SLICES, ROUGHLY CHOPPED

1 TSP CHOPPED FRESH CHIVES

40G GOAT'S FETA (OR ANOTHER VARIETY OF GOAT'S CHEESE), CUT INTO CHUNKS

1 Whisk the eggs in a bowl and season with salt and pepper.

2 Pour a drizzle of oil into a frying pan and place on a medium to high heat. When hot, pour in the eggs and cook on a high heat for 2 minutes, making sure that that the egg mixture is spread out evenly.

3 As the eggs begin to set, lower the heat and add the turkey, chives and goat's feta to one half of the pan.

4 Use a spatula to free the edges, then fold the omelette over and serve.

MUSCLE UP

The protein from the chicken and feta, combined with spinach, helps to speed up the body's conversion of protein into muscle. Remember that rest days are when your body is repairing and rebuilding, so you need an omelette packed with power!

SERVES 1

2 LARGE EGGS

SEA SALT AND FRESHLY
GROUND BLACK PEPPER

COCONUT OR COLD-PRESSED
RAPESEED OIL

2 MINI CHICKEN FILLETS, DICED

50G SPINACH, WASHED

50G GOAT'S MILK FETA

1 Whisk the eggs in a bowl and season with salt and pepper.

2 Pour a drizzle of oil into a frying pan and place on a medium to high heat. Add the chicken, season with salt and pepper, then cook for a few minutes, stirring.

3 When the chicken is cooked thoroughly, stir in the spinach and feta. Cook until the feta has started to melt, then remove to a plate.

4 Wipe the pan with a piece of kitchen paper if necessary, then add a little more oil and return the pan to the heat. Pour in the eggs and cook on a high heat for 2 minutes, making sure that the egg mixture is spread out evenly.

5 As the eggs begin to set, lower the heat and add the chicken, spinach and feta mixture to one half of the pan.

6 Use a spatula to free the edges, then fold the omelette over and serve.

TRAINING DAY BREAKFASTS

Training day breakfasts are all about slow-releasing, high-fibre carbs that will enable you to fuel the slaying of the day! All the recipes here contain quality protein and healthy fats, and I have carefully chosen the suggestions for the porridge add-ins to be high in vitamins and minerals – and to taste great together, of course.

TRAINING DAY BREAKFASTS
MUSHROOM PORRIDGE

Mushrooms are full of protein and fibre, and varieties like shiitake are especially high in selenium, which helps prevent damage to your body's cells as well as supporting your immune system. This savoury porridge – a bit like a quick breakfast risotto – is a different way of incorporating them into your diet. This is the perfect breakfast for people with more of a savoury tooth. If you're pushed for time in the morning, you can soak the mushrooms (steps 1 and 2) the night before. If you're training particularly hard, you could top the porridge with a halved soft-boiled egg, for extra protein.

SERVES 1

A SMALL HANDFUL OF DRIED MUSHROOMS, SUCH AS SHIITAKE OR PORCINI

230ML BOILING WATER

50G JUMBO ROLLED OATS

SEA SALT AND FRESHLY GROUND BLACK PEPPER

A SMALL HANDFUL OF FRESH DILL, CHOPPED

1 Put the mushrooms into a small heatproof bowl and cover with the boiling water. Leave to soak for 20 minutes.

2 Drain the mushrooms, keeping the water they were soaking in, and chop them roughly.

3 Place the oats in a small saucepan with the mushrooms and their soaking water and bring to the boil. Lower the heat and simmer for 3–5 minutes, stirring occasionally.

4 Remove from the heat, season with salt and pepper, and finish with the chopped dill just before eating.

VIKING GRANOLA

Our Viking ancestors had to forage for berries, nuts and seeds. Baking a batch of this granola in advance should make your weekday hunt for breakfast an easier affair! Serve with almond milk or goat's milk yoghurt. If you're pushed for time, pack it into a glass jar or Tupperware for a portable breakfast – just remember, don't eat on the go. Raw honey contains sugar, of course, but it is not heated when processed, which means that it retains its enzymes and nutrients.

MAKES 1 JAR (APPROX. 400G/10–12 PORTIONS)

1½ TBSP COCONUT OIL

1½ TBSP ORGANIC RAW HONEY

100G JUMBO ROLLED OATS

100G RYE FLAKES

20G SUNFLOWER SEEDS

20G PUMPKIN SEEDS

20G HAZELNUTS, ROUGHLY CHOPPED

25G COCONUT FLAKES

SEEDS FROM 6 CARDAMOM PODS, CRUSHED

½ TSP CARAWAY SEEDS, CRUSHED

A PINCH OF SEA SALT

50G DRIED CRANBERRIES OR CHERRIES, CHOPPED

1 Preheat the oven to 140°C/120°C fan/gas 1, and line a baking tray with greaseproof paper.

2 Put the coconut oil and honey into a small pan and melt over a low heat.

3 Mix the oats, rye flakes, seeds, nuts, coconut flakes, spices and salt together in a bowl, then stir in the coconut oil and honey mixture to coat.

4 Spoon the mixture on to the baking tray in an even layer and bake for around 30 minutes, or until golden, giving it a stir every 10 minutes.

5 Remove and leave to cool slightly, then mix in the dried fruit.

PORRIDGE

One of the most versatile of meals, porridge is made for mixing up. I tend to use jumbo oats, but you could also swap in some rye, barley, quinoa or spelt flakes, which have a nutty taste and add a different texture. What makes it so versatile is that you can add different toppings: fresh fruit, nuts, seeds, powders such as cacao and cinnamon, making it impossible to get fed up with it. Below I've given the base recipe and then my favourite toppings and their benefits.

SERVES 1

FOR THE BASE

50G JUMBO ROLLED OATS
(OR 25G JUMBO ROLLED OATS
PLUS 25G RYE, BARLEY,
QUINOA OR SPELT FLAKES)

225ML WATER

A PINCH OF SALT (OPTIONAL)

A SPLASH OF ALMOND OR OAT
MILK (OPTIONAL)

1 Place the oats and water in a small saucepan and bring to the boil. Lower the heat and simmer for 3–5 minutes, stirring. (If you're adding other ingredients such as seeds or ground spices, as in the options below, mix these in now, so the seeds soften and the flavours merge.)

2 Spoon into a bowl, adding a pinch of salt and a splash of milk, if you like, along with any additional toppings, such as fresh fruit or nuts.

IRON ENERGY BOOM

As consumption of red meat has decreased, iron deficiency has become more common. But worry not: iron is found in many foods, and adding these ingredients to your porridge will ensure it is full of it!

1 TBSP RAW UNSWEETENED COCONUT FLAKES OR CHIPS

1 TSP GOJI BERRIES

3 TSBP COCONUT MILK

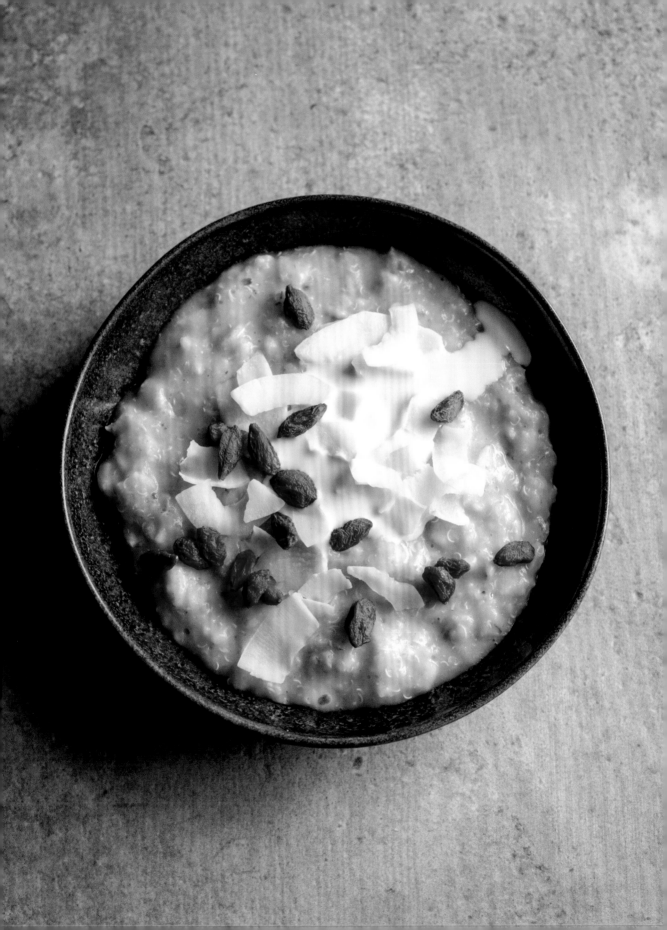

MICRO BOOST

Raspberries and sunflower seeds are a great combination, providing manganese, folate and magnesium, plus vitamins B, C, E and K, which variously help with enzyme and red blood cell production, plus maintaining healthy bones, skin, eyes and blood vessels, among other things, making this option a real micronutrient bomb!

1 TSP SUNFLOWER SEEDS

A HANDFUL OF RASPBERRIES

ANTIOXIDANT SHOT

Full of antioxidants, this is the option to get you geared up and ready to go in your longboat.

1 TSP CACAO POWDER

10 ALMONDS, FINELY CHOPPED, TO SPRINKLE ON TOP

HEART FOOD

Cinnamon is rich in fibre, which helps to maintain good bowel health, and in calcium, which studies suggest protects the heart from blockages, plus the blueberries are shown to help widen arteries.

1 TBSP GROUND CINNAMON

A LARGE HANDFUL OF BLUEBERRIES

IMMUNE INJECTION

Strawberries provide even more vitamin C than oranges, and pumpkin seeds are high in zinc, which improves immunity, is needed for healthy cell division, has a great impact on hormonal balance and aids healthy digestion.

1 TSP PUMPKIN SEEDS

7 STRAWBERRIES, HALVED

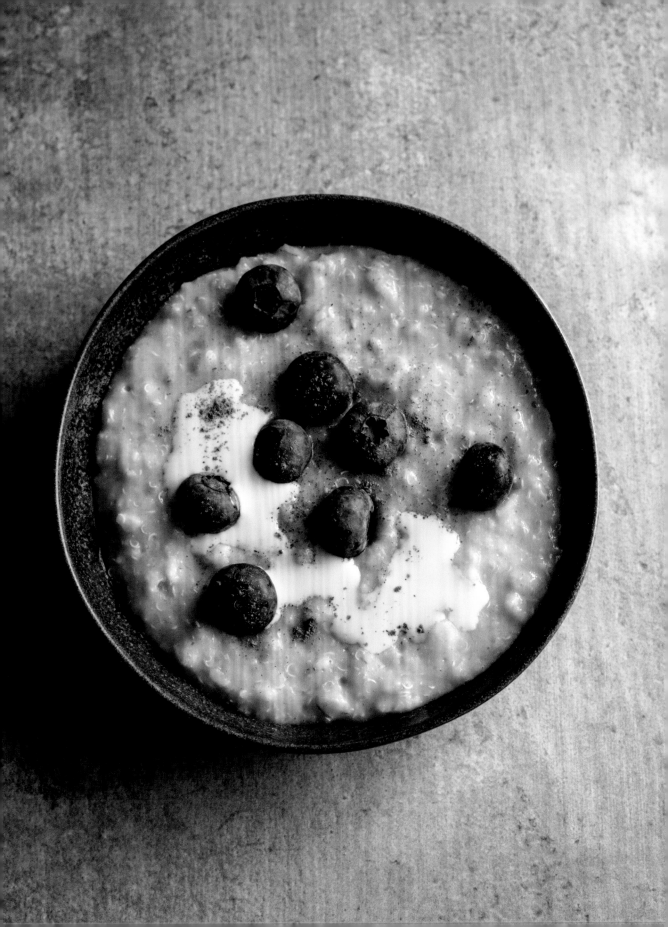

OVERNIGHT CHIA PORRIDGE

An alternative to oats, small black chia seeds swell when soaked, becoming porridge-like in texture. They're high in fibre – 50g should provide about two-thirds of your recommended daily allowance – so they should help to keep you feeling fuller for longer. As you leave this in the fridge overnight, it requires minimal prep first thing, making it great for busy training days and mornings on the go. Mix and match the toppings as with the other porridge recipes (see previous pages).

SERVES 1

50G CHIA SEEDS

250ML ALMOND MILK (OR RICE OR OAT MILK, OR WATER)

1 TSP GROUND CINNAMON

40G BLUEBERRIES

1 Put the chia seeds and almond milk into a bowl and stir.

2 Cover and leave overnight in the fridge.

3 In the morning, stir in the cinnamon, then top with blueberries and enjoy.

BERRY & LIQUORICE CHIA JAM

Frozen berries are just as good for you as fresh, making them a great thing to keep stocked in the freezer. Liquorice root is often used in plant-based medicine for its anti-inflammatory properties, and adds a lovely tangy sweet aniseed flavour here. This fresh jam, thickened by the protein-rich chia seeds, will keep for a week in the fridge. Stir a spoonful through your porridge, or spread it on a slice of toasted Tyr's Post-war Treat (see page 151), dark rye or pumpernickel toast. Berry good!

SERVES 1

450G FROZEN MIXED BERRIES

3 TBSP CHIA SEEDS

1 TSP LIQUORICE ROOT POWDER

1 Put the berries into a pan and place on a medium-low heat, stirring occasionally to help them break down. When defrosted, increase the heat a little to a simmer, then add the chia seeds and liquorice powder and cook for a couple of minutes more, stirring.

2 Remove from the heat and leave to thicken.

BLUEBERRY RYE PANCAKES

SERVES 2

50G RYE FLOUR

50G BUCKWHEAT FLOUR

A PINCH OF SEA SALT

1 EGG

500ML ALMOND MILK

80G BLUEBERRIES

1 TBSP COCONUT OIL

ORGANIC RAW HONEY
(OPTIONAL)

1 Mix the flours, salt, egg and almond milk together in a bowl until fully combined, then leave to rest in the fridge for an hour (or overnight).

2 Remove from the fridge and mix in half the blueberries.

3 Put the coconut oil into a non-stick frying pan over a medium heat. When melted and bubbling, add a couple of spoonfuls of the batter. Cook until golden, then flip and cook the other side. Repeat until the batter is all used up.

4 Serve with the remaining blueberries and a drizzle of raw honey.

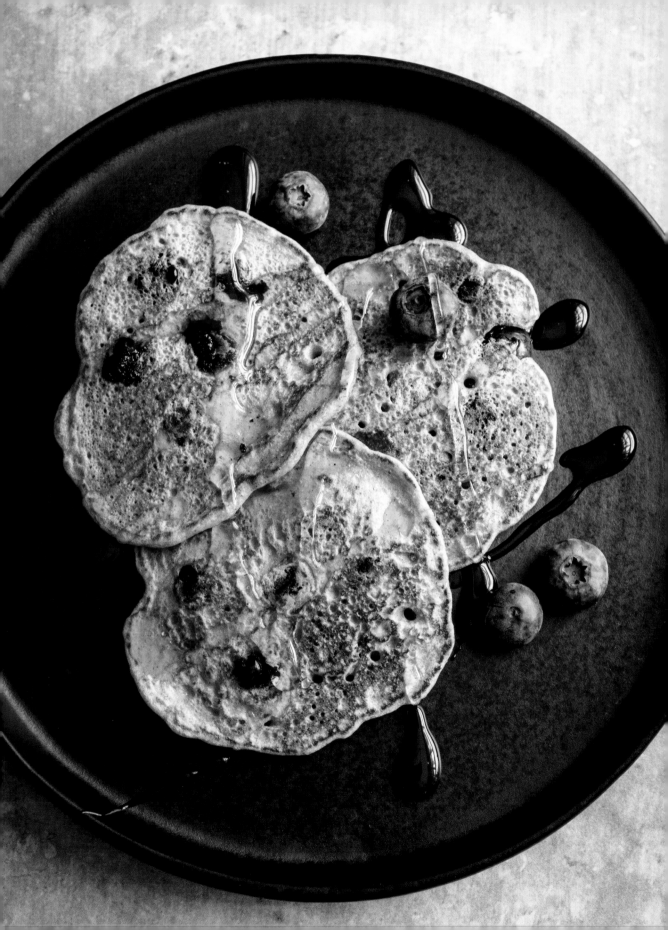

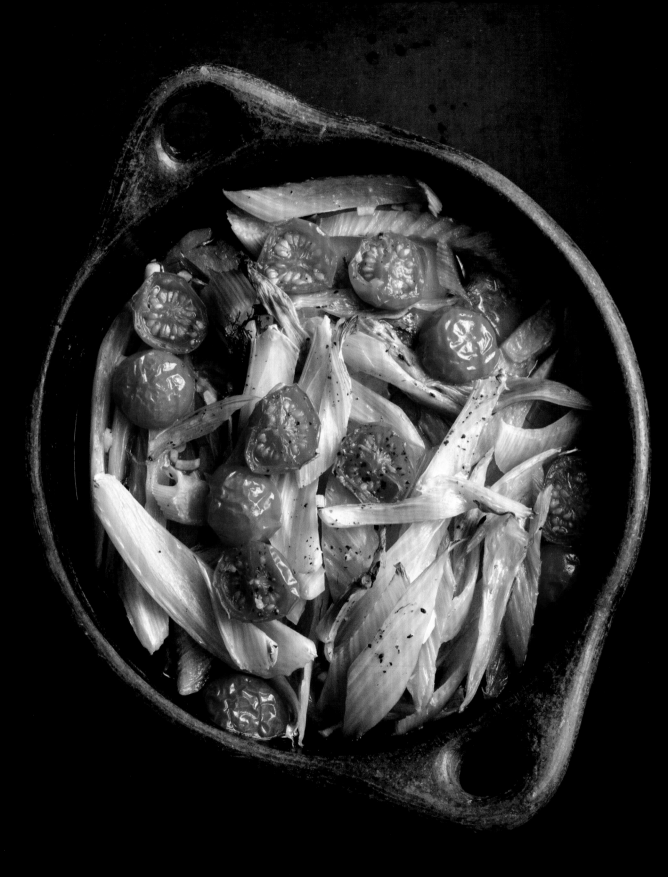

LUNCH AND DINNER

These recipes are divided into:

Post-training Meals – to be eaten after you have worked out. These Post-training Meals work as Anytime Meals. if you just remove the carb element. In their place, add more veggies or one of the Viking Salads (see pages 208–11).

Anytime Meals – to be eaten when you haven't trained before the meal, just add any carb to make them post-workout perfect (see pages 158–90).

POST-TRAINING MEALS

Post-training Meals are meant to be eaten on training days only, after you have worked out. All Post-training Meals include Sometimes Carbs (see pages 11 and 224–9), as it is crucial to replenish your glycogen stores after you train. (Glycogen is stored sugar to be used later. When you train, you use up your glycogen stores in your muscles, which then need to be replenished so that you have energy for your next training session, aka your Viking slaying.) If you can, try to time your Post-training Meal so that you eat within 2 hours of finishing training – this way you will reap the greatest benefits.

All dishes serve one person, unless otherwise stated.

POST-TRAINING MEALS
POTATO AND FENNEL BAKE

This is one of those recipes where time does all the work for you! It's a good one for making ahead if you know you're not going to have time to cook when you get home – just reheat it in the oven for 15 minutes, or until it's warm. Remember, Vikings are always prepared.

SERVES 1

A KNOB OF GOAT'S BUTTER

1 MEDIUM POTATO, PEELED AND THINLY SLICED (AROUND ½CM THICK)

SEA SALT AND FRESHLY GROUND BLACK PEPPER

2 CLOVES OF GARLIC, FINELY CHOPPED

1 SMALL FENNEL BULB, TRIMMED AND THINLY SLICED (AROUND ½CM THICK)

6 CHERRY TOMATOES, HALVED

250ML HOT VEGETABLE STOCK

1 Preheat the oven to 180°C/160°C fan/gas 4.

2 Grease a small ovenproof dish with the butter. Place a layer of potato slices on the bottom of the dish, season with salt and pepper, and dot with garlic. Top with fennel slices, then scatter over a few cherry tomatoes. Repeat until you've used everything up.

3 Pour in the vegetable stock, then cover tightly with foil and bake for around 45 minutes, until crisp and golden.

TIP: If you're not vegetarian, a couple of chopped anchovies dotted among the layers of veg add a delicious salty-savoury flavour.

SPEEDY VIKING SMÖRGÅSBORD

This may seem like a small meal, but it's deceptively filling and ticks all the boxes on the Viking checklist for macro and micro greatness. It's one of my favourites for when I finish training after a long day and want something quick and tasty, without compromising on any health benefits. Add a side salad from the Salad chapter (see pages 206–11) if you like.

SERVES 1

3 MEDIUM EGGS

1 AVOCADO

A SQUEEZE OF LEMON
(OPTIONAL)

SEA SALT AND FRESHLY
GROUND BLACK PEPPER

3 DARK RYE CRACKERS

A FEW SLICES OF PICKLED
SLICED BEETROOT (OPTIONAL)

50G GOAT'S MILK FETA,
CRUMBLED

1 Put the eggs into a pan, fill it with enough cold water to cover them, and place on a medium to high heat. Once boiling, reduce the heat slightly and simmer for 3 minutes, then remove the eggs and place them in a bowl of cold water.

2 Remove the flesh from the avocado and mash it in a bowl. If you want to season it, add a squeeze of lemon and a pinch of salt.

3 Peel and slice the eggs.

4 Spread the mashed avocado over the crackers, then top with the egg, the sliced beetroot, if you are using it, and the crumbled feta, and season with salt and pepper.

SPICY GRAIN BOWL

It's definitely not Icelandic, but even we Vikings know that when hunger strikes and we need to refuel, a burrito never fails. This grain bowl, inspired by typical burrito fillings but without the tortilla wrap element, is quick and easy to put together and full of punchy flavours. Feel free to substitute a diced chicken breast instead of the prawns.

SERVES 1

½ AN AVOCADO

1 LIME

CHILLI FLAKES

SEA SALT

A GENEROUS HANDFUL OF FRESH CORIANDER, CHOPPED

¼ OF A SMALL RED CABBAGE

RED WINE VINEGAR

EXTRA VIRGIN OLIVE OIL

1 TSP COCONUT OIL

150G RAW PRAWNS

1 TSP CAJUN SPICE

1 TSP PAPRIKA

90G COOKED QUINOA (FOLLOW THE INSTRUCTIONS ON THE PACKET)

1 TBSP TOMATO SALSA (SEE PAGE 215 OR USE SHOP-BOUGHT)

1 Scoop the flesh out of the avocado and mash it in a small bowl with a squeeze of lime juice. Add chilli flakes, salt and chopped coriander to taste.

2 Finely slice the red cabbage, and place in a small bowl with a dash of vinegar and olive oil. Mix together to coat the cabbage.

3 Put the coconut oil into a pan on a medium heat. Once hot, add the prawns, Cajun spice and paprika. Stir together, making sure that the prawns are coated. They won't take long to cook – around 3 minutes, or until they turn pink. Make sure you don't overcook them.

4 In a bowl combine the cooked quinoa, prawns, avocado mix, salsa and cabbage. Add a few more coriander leaves for garnish and you are set!

VEGGIE OPTION: You could use 200g of kidney beans or chickpeas instead of the prawns; get organic pre-cooked beans. Put the beans into a pan and heat through. Add to the bowl with all the other ingredients (apart from the prawns, of course), then add Cajun spice and paprika to taste. Another fab veggie option is tofu – 100g, cut into bite-size pieces. Cook in the same way as the prawns, frying for 5 minutes.

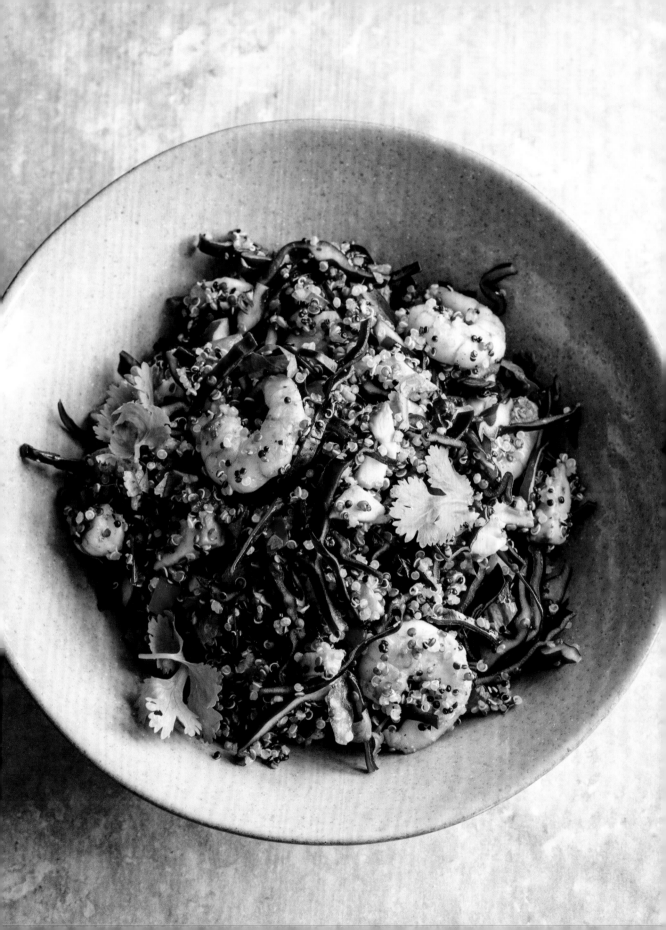

ROAST CHICKEN WITH BABY POTATOES, KIDNEY BEANS & DATES

This is one of my absolute favourite things to eat! The juicy roast chicken mixed with the golden squash and potatoes, and the sweet, crunchy roasted dates topped with tangy melted goat's feta, is a pretty difficult combination to beat.

SERVES 1

1 TSP COCONUT OIL

2 BONE-IN CHICKEN THIGHS

6 BABY NEW POTATOES, CHOPPED IN HALF OR QUARTERED IF THEY ARE LARGER

2 SLICES OF BUTTERNUT SQUASH (AROUND ½CM THICK), CHOPPED INTO CHUNKS

1 CLOVE OF GARLIC, CHOPPED

½ A RED PEPPER, DESEEDED AND DICED

1–2 TOMATOES, QUARTERED

SEA SALT AND FRESHLY GROUND BLACK PEPPER

150G TINNED KIDNEY BEANS

50G GOAT'S MILK FETA, CHOPPED INTO CHUNKS

3 DATES, PITTED AND HALVED

1 Preheat the oven to 200°C/180°C fan/gas 6 and grease a roasting tray with the coconut oil.

2 Place the chicken thighs, potatoes and squash in the tray and put into the oven. Roast for 20 minutes, until golden and starting to crisp, then add the garlic, red pepper and tomatoes and season with salt and pepper.

3 Cook for a further 15 minutes, then add the kidney beans, feta and dates. When the beans are a bit split and the feta is melted, it's ready to eat.

SPICY BEANS OR CHICKPEAS

These warmly spiced beans are fantastic: they improve cardiovascular health, are high in antioxidants and fibre, improve digestion, give long-lasting energy and taste so good. Serve them warm with rice or quinoa (see Sometimes Carbs, pages 224–9), cold with salad (see Salads, pages 206–11), or as an accompaniment to grilled chicken or steak. It's worth doubling the quantities to have leftovers!

SERVES 1

100G DRIED BLACK TURTLE BEANS OR CHICKPEAS, SOAKED OVERNIGHT (OR USE TINNED BEANS)

1 TSP COCONUT OIL

½ TSP CUMIN SEEDS

1 MEDIUM TOMATO, CHOPPED

2–3CM PIECE OF FRESH GINGER, PEELED AND GRATED

½ TSP GROUND TURMERIC

1 TSP GROUND CORIANDER

1 TSP SEA SALT

¼ TSP CHILLI POWDER (OPTIONAL)

FRESHLY GROUND BLACK PEPPER

1 Soak the dried black turtle beans or chickpeas overnight (or for at least 8 hours) – if you're using tinned beans then of course there is no need to soak them, just drain and add them to the pan in step 5.

2 Drain the soaked beans or chickpeas and rinse in fresh water. Then put into a pan with 500ml of water. Bring to the boil, then reduce the heat and simmer for an hour.

3 Put the coconut oil into a pan on a high heat. When hot, add the cumin seeds – when you hear them start to crackle, add the tomato and ginger, lower the heat slightly to medium, and stir together.

4 Add the turmeric, coriander and salt to the pan and cook, stirring occasionally, for 3–4 minutes. If the mixture starts to stick, add a splash of water to loosen it.

5 Add the beans or chickpeas and the chilli powder, if using. Stir all together for 2–3 minutes and you are done.

6 Season with salt and pepper to taste.

PESTO CHICKEN & SWEET POTATO ONE-TRAY WONDER

My mum created this recipe and it has become a weekly regular for me and my daughter, Raven! It is absolutely delicious.

SERVES 2

1 TSP COCONUT OIL

2 SMALL TO MEDIUM SWEET POTATOES

SEA SALT AND FRESHLY GROUND BLACK PEPPER

3–4 MINI CHICKEN BREAST FILLETS

2 TBSP KALE & WALNUT PESTO (SEE PAGE 215)

70G GOAT'S MILK FETA, CHOPPED FINELY

185G TINNED KIDNEY BEANS, DRAINED

70G KALE, WASHED AND DRIED, RIPPED INTO SMALL PIECES

1 Preheat the oven to 200°C/180°C fan/gas 6 and grease a roasting tray with the coconut oil.

2 Peel the sweet potatoes, or scrub them with a vegetable brush, and cut them into chips. Arrange the chips in the roasting tray, season with salt and pepper, and put into the oven to cook for 15 minutes.

3 Remove the tray from the oven and turn the chips so they cook evenly. Create some space in the tray and add the chicken fillets. Brush a thick layer of pesto over the chicken, then crumble over the feta. Put the tray back into the oven and cook for another 20–25 minutes. The sweet potato should be soft and coloured at the edges and the chicken cooked through but still juicy. (Slice into the thickest part to check, if you are unsure – the meat should be white and the juices clear.)

4 About 5 minutes before the chicken and chips are ready, add the kidney beans and the kale to the tray, mixing everything together (without disturbing the chips too much) and seasoning again.

5 Serve straight from the oven.

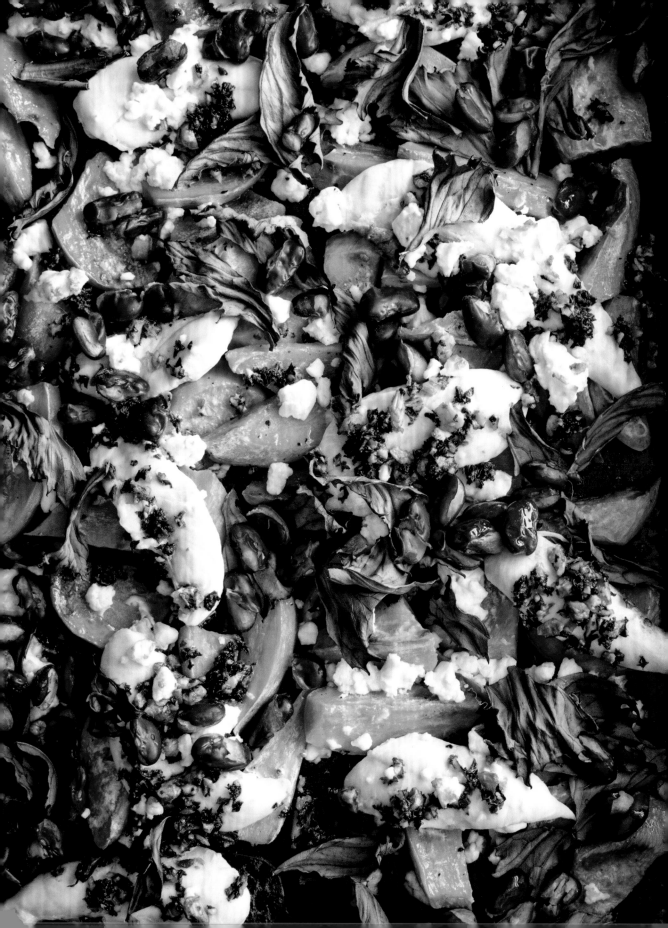

BUTTERY SALMON WITH PAPRIKA RICE

Adding goat's butter to the salmon really enhances its rich flavour – it's one of my favourite fast-track tips to a super tasty meal.

SERVES 1

1 TSP COCONUT OIL, OR COLD-PRESSED RAPESEED OIL

100G BROWN RICE

500ML WATER

2 TSP PAPRIKA

1–2 SALMON FILLETS

A GOOD KNOB OF GOAT'S MILK BUTTER, OR VEGAN BUTTER

SEA SALT AND FRESHLY GROUND BLACK PEPPER

1 SHALLOT, QUARTERED

½ A COURGETTE, CHOPPED

½ A RED OR YELLOW PEPPER, DESEEDED AND CHOPPED

1 Preheat the oven to 200°C/180°C fan/gas 6. Line a roasting tray with tin foil and spread the oil over it.

2 Rinse the rice, then drain and put into a pan. Pour over the water and bring to the boil, then lower the heat to a simmer, cover the pan and cook according to the packet instructions (these can vary). When done, drain the rice and stir in the paprika. Cover the pan and leave to sit.

3 While the rice is cooking, place the salmon in the roasting tray, coat with the butter and season with salt and pepper. Add the shallot, then put the tray into the oven and roast for 10 minutes.

4 Add the courgettes and peppers and put back into the oven for a further 10 minutes.

5 Serve the buttery salmon and vegetables on top of the paprika rice.

CHICKEN WITH CURRIED SCRAMBLED EGGS, LENTILS & GOOD STUFF

With garlic, ginger and beetroot – aka the Good Stuff – this is a proper energy and wellness boost, and packed full of flavour!

SERVES 1

100G GREEN LENTILS

400ML WATER

2 MEDIUM EGGS

1 TSP COCONUT OIL

1 LARGE CHICKEN BREAST, DICED

1 CLOVE OF GARLIC, CHOPPED

2–3CM PIECE OF FRESH GINGER, PEELED AND GRATED

½ A CHICKEN STOCK CUBE, DISSOLVED IN 100ML WATER

1–2 TBSP CURRY POWDER, TO TASTE

1 COOKED BEETROOT, SLICED

50G GOAT'S MILK FETA, CUT INTO CUBES

50G SPINACH, WASHED

SEA SALT AND FRESHLY GROUND BLACK PEPPER

1 Rinse the lentils in a sieve, then put into a pan with the water. Bring to the boil, then reduce the heat and simmer for 15–20 minutes, or until the lentils are tender. Drain immediately.

2 Crack the eggs into a bowl and whisk together. Stir in the cooked lentils and set aside.

3 Put the coconut oil into a pan and place on a medium heat. When hot, add the chicken and cook for about 7 minutes, stirring occasionally, until cooked through.

4 Add the garlic and ginger, and cook for a minute to soften.

5 Add the egg and lentil mixture to the pan, along with the chicken stock, curry powder and sliced beetroot. Stir continuously until the eggs begin to scramble.

6 Just before the eggs are fully cooked, add the feta and spinach and season with salt and pepper. Cook for a minute or so more, until the spinach wilts.

7 Remove from the heat immediately and spoon into a bowl.

VEGGIE OPTION: This dish works just as well without the chicken – add an extra egg if you like.

ICELANDIC LAMB STEW

This dish has been with us Vikings for a long time. It's perfect for cold winter evenings, as it warms up the soul and energizes and strengthens the body.

SERVES 2–3

1 TSP COCONUT OIL, OR COLD-PRESSED RAPESEED OIL

500G LAMB RUMP, CUT INTO CHUNKS

1 LITRE WATER

½ A BEEF STOCK CUBE

1 ONION, FINELY CHOPPED

1 STALK OF CELERY, CHOPPED

1 CARROT, ROUGHLY CHOPPED

1 SWEDE, ROUGHLY CHOPPED

100G BROWN RICE, RINSED

5 DROPS OF TABASCO SAUCE

SEA SALT AND FRESHLY GROUND BLACK PEPPER

FRESH DILL, CHOPPED

1 Put the oil into a casserole or a heavy-bottomed saucepan and place on a medium-high heat. When hot, add the chunks of lamb but don't overcrowd the pan – you can cook the meat in batches if you need to. The lamb should sizzle as it hits the pan. Cook until browned, repeating as necessary and removing each batch to a plate.

2 Put all the lamb back into the pan along with the rest of the ingredients, except the dill. Bring to the boil, then reduce the heat to a simmer, cover and cook for 30 minutes. Give it a stir and season with salt and pepper.

3 Serve with the fresh dill sprinkled on top.

ALL-THE-GREENS SPELTOTTO

SERVES 2

2 TSP COLD-PRESSED
RAPESEED OIL

1 SHALLOT, FINELY CHOPPED

SEA SALT AND FRESHLY
GROUND BLACK PEPPER

100G PEARLED SPELT

8 BROCCOLI FLORETS,
CHOPPED INTO SMALL PIECES

250ML VEGETABLE STOCK

3 TBSP KALE & WALNUT PESTO
(SEE PAGE 215)

1 Put the oil into a pan and place on a medium heat. When hot, add the shallot and a pinch of salt and cook for a couple of minutes, until soft.

2 Add the spelt and cook for a couple more minutes, stirring constantly to prevent it sticking and to ensure it's coated with the oil and shallots. Add the broccoli and cook for a minute more, stirring.

3 Reduce the heat to medium-low, then add enough stock to just cover everything, stirring to combine. Cook the speltotto for around 10 minutes, adding more stock as needed until it is all absorbed and the spelt is just cooked – it should still have a little bite to it.

4 Stir in the pesto, and continue cooking for a couple more minutes. Add a splash of water if necessary – it should have the consistency of risotto. Taste and adjust the seasoning to your liking before serving.

THE WARRIOR PASTA SALAD

This is such a perfect post-workout meal, as it's super-quick and simple to put together – an advantage when you are absolutely dead from smashing your training! It's all about powering through.

SERVES 1

SEA SALT AND FRESHLY GROUND BLACK PEPPER

100G WHOLEWHEAT PASTA

1 TSP COCONUT OIL, OR COLD-PRESSED RAPESEED OIL

1 LARGE CHICKEN BREAST, CUT INTO BITE-SIZE PIECES

250G GOAT'S MILK YOGHURT

1 TSP CAJUN SPICE

½ A RED PEPPER, DESEEDED AND CHOPPED

½ AN ONION, FINELY CHOPPED

4 CAULIFLOWER FLORETS

1 CARROT, PEELED AND ROUGHLY CHOPPED

>> SAY NO TO LOW
Fat has flavour. Cereals, yoghurts, snack bars and ready meals proclaiming to be 'low-fat' on their packaging are not healthy. It follows that, as some of the fat has been removed, it's been replaced with something else. More often than not, this is sugar. A LOT of sugar. So put the low-fat down and pick up the full-fat! It tastes better, and it's better for you too.

1 Bring a pot of water to the boil. When it's bubbling, add salt and then the pasta. Cook according to the instructions on the packet, then drain and leave to cool.

2 While the pasta is cooking, put the oil into a pan and place on a medium heat. When hot, add the chicken and stir-fry for around 7 minutes, or until cooked through, stirring occasionally. Remove from the heat and leave to cool.

3 Put the yoghurt into a medium-size bowl and mix with the Cajun spice.

4 Add the cooked pasta and chicken along with the other ingredients, mixing together so that everything is coated in the spiced yoghurt. Season to taste with salt and pepper, and serve.

VEGGIE OPTION: Roast 150g of tinned chickpeas for 30 minutes at 200°C/180°C fan/gas 6. (Coat the chickpeas with coconut oil and place on a foil-lined baking tray, then season with salt and pepper and go! When crisp, remove from the oven, leave to cool, then add to the salad.)

PESCATARIAN OPTION: Replace the chicken with a hot smoked trout fillet, broken up into flakes, or 100g of cooked king prawns, and swap the Cajun spice for a generous handful of chopped fresh dill.

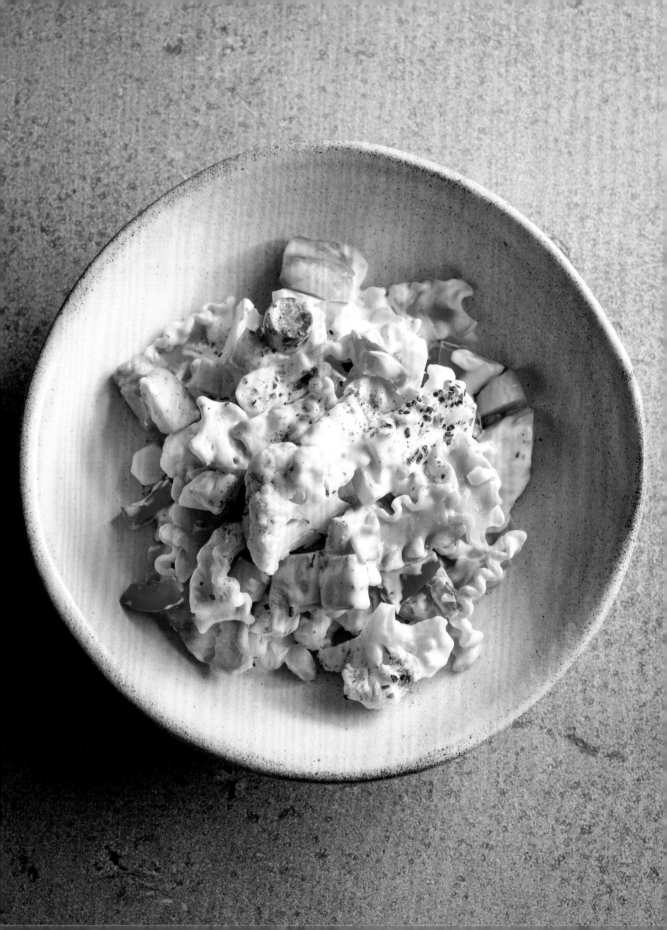

BEETROOT & CHICKPEA DISCS

Quick to make, easy to pack up and take with you: healthy fast food! These are perfect to have with chicken breast (diced, then grilled in a pan for 8–10 minutes), as a burger or with one of the salads (see pages 206–11). Any leftover discs will keep in the fridge for up to 3 days.

MAKES 6 DISCS (ENOUGH FOR 2–3)

1 x 400G TIN OF ORGANIC CHICKPEAS, DRAINED

90G COOKED BEETROOT

50G GOAT'S MILK FETA

4 SPRING ONIONS

PAPRIKA

SEA SALT AND FRESHLY GROUND BLACK PEPPER

1 TSP COCONUT OIL

1 Put the chickpeas into a bowl and mash them.

2 Chop the beetroot, feta and spring onions finely and add to the bowl with paprika, salt and pepper to taste. Mix together so everything is evenly distributed.

3 Scoop out a tablespoonful and roll between your hands – it should be like a big golfball. Flatten out into a disc shape. Repeat with the rest of the mixture.

4 Put the coconut oil into a pan on a high heat. When the oil has melted and the pan is hot, lower the heat to medium and add the discs.

5 Cook until golden brown and crisping underneath, about 2 minutes, then flip (a spatula or fish slice is handy here) and repeat on the other side. Remove to a plate lined with kitchen paper to drain before eating.

KING PRAWNS IN BLACK RICE

Black rice is high in antioxidants, rich in anti-inflammatories, and great for liver and heart health as well as cognitive function. Ancient Chinese tales suggest it was forbidden to anyone other than the Emperor and the Royal Family because of its nutritional properties and healing powers. Luckily for us, those times are gone!

SERVES 1

70G BLACK RICE

1 TSP COCONUT OIL

140G PEELED RAW PRAWNS

30G FROZEN PEAS

1 TSP CHILLI POWDER

1 TSP GROUND CORIANDER

½ A SMALL CARROT,
CUT INTO MATCHSTICKS

½ A RED PEPPER, DESEEDED
AND CHOPPED

SEA SALT AND FRESHLY
GROUND BLACK PEPPER

JUICE OF 1 LIME

1 Put the rice into a colander and rinse two or three times, until the water runs clear. Place in a pan with 140ml of water. Bring to the boil, then reduce the heat and simmer until the water has been absorbed, around 25–35 minutes. Turn off the heat and leave the rice in the pan for 10 minutes.

2 Put the coconut oil into a pan and place on a high heat. Once the oil has melted and the pan is hot, add the prawns, peas, chilli and coriander. Cook, stirring for a minute, then add the carrot and red pepper. Cook for another 2 minutes, continuing to stir, then add the rice. Mix everything together and cook for a couple more minutes, until the prawns are completely pink and the rice is piping hot. Season with salt and pepper, and squeeze over the lime juice before serving.

DATES WRAPPED IN BACON WITH STUFFED MUSHROOM

Every time I have this dish, it feels like I am being rewarded for something extraordinary that I did. I don't always know what it is, but I'll take the reward!

SERVES 1

½ TSP COCONUT OIL

8 PITTED DRIED DATES

4 RASHERS OF STREAKY BACON, HALVED

1 LARGE PORTOBELLO MUSHROOM

100G TINNED KIDNEY BEANS, DRAINED

½ AN AVOCADO

1 Preheat the oven to 220°C/200°C fan/gas 7.

2 Line a roasting tray with foil and grease it with the coconut oil.

3 Wrap each date in half a piece of bacon and secure with a toothpick. Place in the roasting tray and bake in the oven for around 6 minutes, or until the bacon is crisp.

4 While the dates are in the oven, remove the stalk from the mushroom and place the kidney beans in the mushroom cap.

5 Turn the dates over so they will crisp evenly, and add the mushroom to the tray. Return it to the oven and cook for another 6 minutes, then remove.

6 Slice the avocado and add to the mushroom and dates. Plate everything up and enjoy!

VEGGIE OPTION: Try substituting strips of smoky tempeh or vegan bacon – or use a mandolin to peel a courgette into long ribbons and wrap these around the dates.

COD WITH PINEAPPLE & BROWN RICE

Vikings were, and still are, known for being massive fish-eaters. I am lucky in that I love the taste of fish, but whether it's your favourite or not, if you are able to incorporate it into your diet, the health benefits are too substantial not to. Current guidelines recommend eating at least two portions of fish a week (with one of those being an oily variety). Research suggests that different varieties of fish may respectively preserve heart health, improve brain and immune function, and boost the health and appearance of skin and hair. This recipe is one of my mother's crazy creations and pairs delicate cod with savoury nutty brown rice and sweet pineapple. She loves trying out new things and using up anything in the fridge: there's never any food waste in her house! Because she is a fantastic chef, she manages to combine things that you would never think of putting together, but that actually work incredibly well, like fish and fruit.

SERVES 2

100G BROWN RICE

SEA SALT AND LEMON PEPPER

2 SKINLESS BONELESS COD FILLETS (APPROX. 300G)

1 TSP COCONUT OIL

100G CLOSED-CUP MUSHROOMS, SLICED

1 HEAPED TBSP TINNED PINEAPPLE CHUNKS

1 TUB (APPROX. 150G) SHEEP'S MILK YOGHURT

2 TSP CURRY POWDER

100ML PINEAPPLE JUICE (FROM THE TINNED PINEAPPLE)

125G BUFFALO MOZZARELLA

1 Put the brown rice into a pan with 500ml of water and a pinch of salt. Bring to the boil, then reduce the heat and let it simmer for 35 minutes. Drain.

2 Preheat the oven to 200°C/180°C fan/gas 6. Line a roasting tray with foil.

3 When the oven is hot, place the cod in the tray and roast in the oven for 5 minutes. Remove, then carefully slide the cod on to a plate using a fish slice or spatula, and pour any liquid off the tray. Add the coconut oil to the tray, spoon the rice evenly over its surface and place the fish back on top of the rice. Dot the mushrooms and pineapple chunks over the fish and rice, and season with salt and lemon pepper.

4 In a small bowl, mix together the yoghurt, curry powder and pineapple juice and pour over the cod and rice. Finally, cut the cheese into small pieces and dot evenly over everything.

5 Decrease the oven to 180°C/160°C fan/gas 4 and roast for another 25 minutes, until the mozzarella is golden.

CHILLI KING PRAWNS WITH FRIED RICE

Prawns are rich in protein, omega-3, vitamin E, B vitamins and zinc. They also contain astaxanthin, which can act as a potent antioxidant and is anti-inflammatory. Fried rice is best made using rice boiled a couple of days previously and left in the fridge (as this dries it out slightly). You can still make it with just-cooked rice but the texture will be a bit more sticky.

SERVES 1

140G COOKED ORGANIC KING PRAWNS, PEELED

1 TSP CHILLI FLAKES

A SMALL HANDFUL OF FRESH CORIANDER (LEAVES AND STALKS), CHOPPED

JUICE OF ½ A LEMON

100G COOKED LONG-GRAIN WHITE RICE

1 TSP COCONUT OIL

1 LARGE EGG, WHISKED

4 SPRING ONIONS, SLICED

6 BROCCOLI FLORETS

50G FROZEN PEAS

70G BABY SPINACH, WASHED

A DRIZZLE OF SOY SAUCE

1 Put the prawns, chilli flakes and coriander into a medium-size bowl and squeeze over the lemon juice. Leave to marinate while you prepare the rest of the ingredients.

2 Decant the rice into a second medium-size bowl.

3 Put ½ teaspoon of coconut oil into a pan large enough to hold all the ingredients without being too crowded, and place on a medium heat. When the oil is melted and the pan is hot, add the egg, leave for a second, then stir with a wooden spoon until lightly scrambled. Remove from the heat and add to the bowl of rice.

4 Add the remaining oil to the pan and, when hot, cook the spring onions for a minute or two, until just softening. Next, add the prawns, making sure to scrape in all their marinade (a spatula is handy here). Cook for a couple of minutes, stirring, until completely pink and cooked through. Remove from the pan and add to the bowl of rice and egg.

5 Add the broccoli and peas and cook for 2–3 minutes – they should be tender but still with a bit of crunch. When they're almost there, stir in the spinach and cook until just wilted. Now add the rice mixture to the pan, stirring to combine. Cook for a few minutes, stirring all the time: the rice should be piping hot when served. Plate up and add soy sauce to taste.

VEGGIE OPTION: Smoked firm tofu is delicious in place of the prawns – just cut it into bite-size pieces and fry gently until evenly browned before adding to the rice.

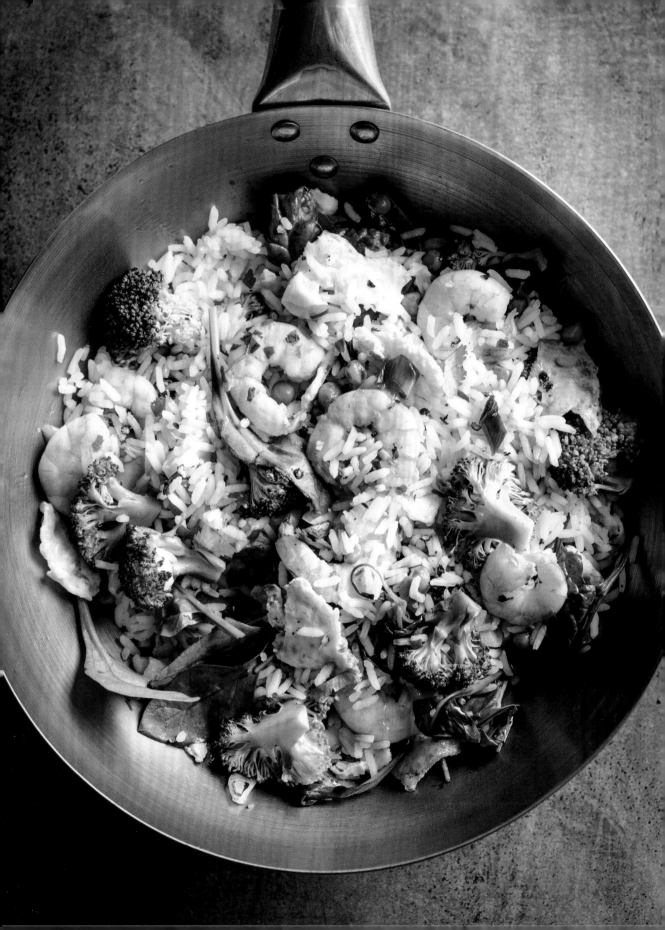

HEARTY HERBY COD WITH SWEET SWEDE MASH

Swede mash is a dish that reminds me of my childhood, although in those days quite a lot of sugar would be mixed in! Swede mash is such a typical Icelandic side dish, common with fish or lamb. Now I add that pop of sweetness with raisins, which contain B vitamins, iron and potassium.

SERVES 1

1 SWEDE, PEELED AND DICED

SEA SALT AND FRESHLY GROUND BLACK PEPPER

A SMALL HANDFUL OF RAISINS, TO TASTE

GROUND CINNAMON, TO TASTE

1 TSP COCONUT OIL, OR COLD-PRESSED RAPESEED OIL

1 SKINLESS BONELESS COD FILLET (APPROX. 150G)

40G SHEEP'S BUTTER, CUT INTO SMALL PIECES

A SPLASH OF WHITE WINE

A LARGE HANDFUL OF FRESH HERBS: BASIL, CORIANDER, CHIVES, DILL, PARSLEY, TARRAGON, CHOPPED

JUICE OF ½ A LEMON

1 Preheat the oven to 180°C/160°C fan/gas 4.

2 Put the swede into a pan with enough cold water to just cover it and a generous pinch of salt. Place on a medium to high heat and bring to the boil, then reduce the heat to a low simmer. Cook for 15 minutes or until tender. (If a small knife slides smoothly in and comes out without any swede on it, it's ready.) Drain, then return it to the pan and mash. Add the raisins and the cinnamon (I generally use 2 teaspoons, but add a little first, then taste and adjust as you like). Cover and keep warm.

3 While the swede is cooking, line a roasting tray with enough foil to cover the cod, and spread the coconut oil over it. Place the cod in the tray, dot over the butter and splash over the wine. Season with salt and pepper, sprinkle over the herbs and lemon juice, then fold the foil over the cod and roast for 15 minutes, or until hot and fully cooked through.

4 Serve alongside the swede mash.

TIP: Adding butter to mash is always yummy and gives it an even more intensely creamy, rich flavour. If raisins and cinnamon aren't your thing, instead try mixing additional finely chopped herbs through the mash (a good way to ensure they don't go to waste), or a heaped teaspoon of Dijon mustard. Mix up your mash.

ARCTIC CHAR WITH APPLES & RED ONION

Arctic char is a cold-water fish that's part of the trout and salmon family. It's a great source of protein, low in mercury, high in omega-3s and incredibly popular in Iceland, though it's less well known in the UK. You might be thinking: fish and fruit? But trust me. The combination of the savoury char and the sweet apple is magic. And of course, adding butter makes it even better.

SERVES 1

100G BROWN RICE

SEA SALT AND FRESHLY GROUND BLACK PEPPER

1 LEMON

1 TSP COCONUT OIL

1 ARCTIC CHAR FILLET (APPROX. 120G)

1 ROYAL GALA APPLE

1 MEDIUM RED ONION

40G SHEEP'S BUTTER

1 SMALL BUNCH OF FRESH PARSLEY, FINELY CHOPPED

1 Preheat the oven to 180°C/160°C fan/gas 4.

2 Put the brown rice into a pan with 500ml of water and a pinch of salt. Bring to the boil, then reduce the heat and let it simmer for 35 minutes. Drain.

3 Zest the lemon into a small bowl until you have about a teaspoonful, then sprinkle in some sea salt and rub together with your fingers so that the fragrant citrus oil infuses the salt.

4 Line a roasting tray with foil and spread the coconut oil over it, then place the fish in the middle.

5 Cut the apple and red onion into eighths (in quarters, then halve each quarter), and lay them around the fish. Dot with the butter and season everything with the lemon salt and pepper. Sprinkle over half the parsley and roast in the oven for 15 minutes, or until hot and fully cooked through.

6 Serve the char, apple and onion with the rice and sprinkle over the remaining parsley.

TIP: It's easy to make your own flavoured salts, and these are a speedy, sure-fire route to adding an extra punch of flavour to even the simplest cooked fish and vegetables. Lemon zest is a classic, but lime zest works well too (especially with Asian-inspired recipes), as do sturdier herbs like regular or lemon thyme and rosemary – just finely chop the leaves, or grate the zest and rub into the salt (really work it in!) to infuse.

LEMONY SALMON WITH EGG NOODLES

Known for their therapeutic properties throughout the ages, lemons help to strengthen your immune system, aid in blood purifying and cleanse your stomach. I like to squeeze lemon juice into water, over salads and over fish, such as this fantastic salmon.

SERVES 1

140G SALMON FILLET

1 TSP FRESH OREGANO

SEA SALT AND FRESHLY GROUND BLACK PEPPER

1 LEMON, HALVED

1 NEST OF EGG NOODLES

50G FINE GREEN BEANS, ENDS TRIMMED AND CUT IN HALF

6 BROCCOLI FLORETS, CUT INTO BITE-SIZE PIECES

1 TSP COCONUT OIL

4 SPRING ONIONS, CHOPPED

2 CLOVES OF GARLIC, FINELY CHOPPED

1 SMALL RED CHILLI, DESEEDED AND FINELY CHOPPED

2 TSP POMEGRANATE SEEDS

1 Preheat the oven to 200°C/180°C fan/gas 6.

2 Line a roasting tray with a piece of foil large enough to cover the salmon. Place the salmon in the middle, sprinkle with the oregano, season with salt and pepper and squeeze the lemon juice over the top. Fold the foil over the salmon and cook in the oven for 15 minutes. Remove and check that the fish is cooked through (give it a couple of minutes more if not), then break into bite-size pieces.

3 While the salmon is cooking, put a pan of water on to boil and cook the noodles according to the instructions on the packet. Add the green beans and broccoli for the final 3 minutes. Drain and transfer to a bowl.

4 Put the coconut oil into a pan on a medium heat. When the oil is melted and the pan is hot, add the spring onions and garlic and stir-fry for a minute. Add the chilli and stir-fry for another minute. Finally, add the noodles, broccoli, green beans and the salmon, folding everything together carefully (try not to break up the salmon too much) to ensure it heats evenly. Cook for around 4 minutes, or until everything is hot. Season with salt and pepper, sprinkle over the pomegranate seeds and serve.

VEGGIE OPTION: Roast half an aubergine instead of the salmon. Trim the ends and cut into 1cm-thick finger-shaped pieces. Place in a foil-lined roasting tray and rub with a drizzle of rapeseed oil, then squeeze over the lemon, season with salt and pepper and sprinkle over the oregano. Roast, uncovered, for around 25 minutes, or until totally soft.

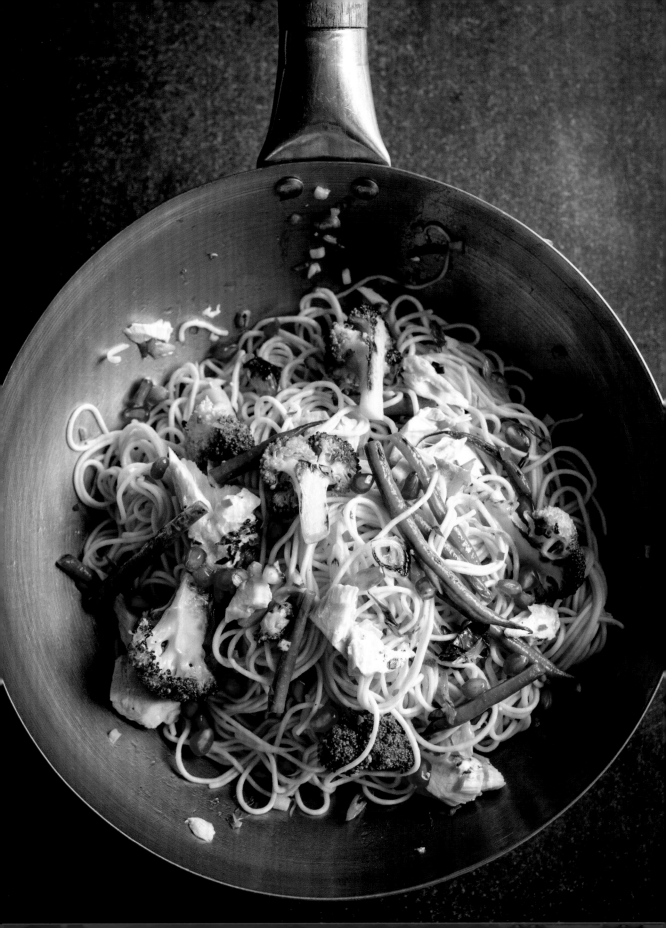

STEAK WITH CINNAMON-SPICED SWEET POTATO MASH

If you've never tried adding cinnamon to your sweet potato mash, then you are in for a massive treat! With protein, healthy fats, slow-releasing carbs, and a dash of antioxidant and anti-inflammatory properties for good measure, it's a proper Viking mash up!

SERVES 1

40G PUMPKIN SEEDS

SEA SALT AND FRESHLY GROUND BLACK PEPPER

SIRLOIN STEAK (APPROX. 250G, AROUND 3CM THICK)

A DRIZZLE OF COLD-PRESSED RAPESEED OIL

70G SPINACH, WASHED

½ AN AVOCADO, PEELED AND SLICED

50G GOAT'S MILK FETA, CUT INTO CHUNKS

A DRIZZLE OF EXTRA VIRGIN OLIVE OIL

A SQUEEZE OF LEMON JUICE

FOR THE MASH

1 LARGE SWEET POTATO, PEELED AND CHOPPED

SEA SALT

1 TBSP GROUND CINNAMON

A DASH OF SHEEP'S, OAT OR SOYA MILK

1 To make the sweet potato mash, put the potatoes into a pot with enough water to cover and a pinch of salt if you like. Put on a medium heat and simmer until soft, about 15–20 minutes (stick a knife in to check if you're not sure – when it slides through, it's ready).

2 Remove from the heat and mash immediately, adding the cinnamon and a splash of milk and seasoning with salt. It won't be completely smooth but should have a good creamy texture.

3 While the potato is cooking, put a small frying pan on a low to medium heat. When hot, add the pumpkin seeds and cook for a few minutes, keeping an eye on them and stirring the pan occasionally. As soon as they start to turn brown and pop (you should be able to smell them), remove from the heat, seasoning with salt. Leave to cool.

4 Rub the steak with the rapeseed oil and season on both sides. Put a frying pan on a medium-high heat. When hot (you want it really hot), put the steak into the pan. I like steak medium rare, so I cook it for 3–4 minutes on each side. If you want it rarer or more well done, adjust the cooking time accordingly (around 2–3 minutes for rare, and 5–6 minutes for well done, though of course this will depend on the thickness of your steak). When cooked to your liking, remove the steak to a plate or board and leave to rest.

5 Put the spinach, avocado, feta and toasted pumpkin seeds into a medium bowl with a small drizzle of olive oil and a squeeze of lemon juice. Mix together with your hands gently, so that everything is coated.

6 Put the steak on a plate with the yummy cinnamon mash, and serve the salad in a side bowl. Boom.

SIRLOIN STEAK WITH PARSNIP FRIES

Parsnips are high in fibre and contain a wide range of vitamins and minerals. They are excellent as chips and go well with chicken, turkey and fish, but they are best with a nice, juicy sirloin steak!

SERVES 1

2 MEDIUM PARSNIPS

3 TSP COLD-PRESSED RAPESEED OIL

SEA SALT AND FRESHLY GROUND BLACK PEPPER

1 TSP GARLIC SALT

CHILLI FLAKES, TO TASTE

1 SHALLOT, FINELY CHOPPED

2 TBSP OLIVE OIL

2 TBSP DIJON MUSTARD

1 TBSP RED WINE VINEGAR

1 SIRLOIN STEAK (APPROX. 250G, AROUND 3CM THICK)

1 Preheat the oven to 200°C/180°C fan/gas 6. Peel the parsnips or scrub with a vegetable brush, then cut them lengthways into long thin wedges, like fries. They don't have to be perfect – the more wonkily they're cut, the better they'll taste.

2 Line a roasting tray with foil. Put the parsnips in the tray, drizzle over 2 teaspoons of rapeseed oil, and season with salt and pepper, the garlic salt and chilli flakes. Mix together with your hands, making sure the parsnips get nicely coated, and roast for 20–30 minutes, turning once halfway through, until they are crisp and caramelized at the edges and soft and juicy within.

3 Put the shallot, olive oil, mustard, vinegar and a little salt and pepper into a food processor and blitz briefly, stopping as soon as it reaches a thick sauce-like consistency.

4 Rub the steak with the remaining rapeseed oil and season on both sides with salt and pepper. Put a frying pan on a medium-high heat. When hot (you want it really hot), put the steak into the pan. I like steak medium rare, so I cook it for 3–4 minutes on each side. If you want it rarer or more well done, adjust the cooking time accordingly (around 2–3 minutes for rare, and 5–6 minutes for well done, though of course this will depend on the thickness of your steak). When cooked to your liking, remove the steak from the heat to a plate or board and leave to rest.

5 Place the steak on a plate with the parsnips and serve with the sauce alongside.

SEABASS, BIFRÖST VEG & RICE

Bifröst is the burning rainbow in Norse mythology that reaches from Midgard, where humans live, to Asgard, where the Gods live. The veggies and spices in this recipe come in the colours of the rainbow, hence the name! Different colours give different goodness, so we are getting extreme greatness in this wonderful recipe. We are off to Asgard!

SERVES 1

100G BROWN RICE

500ML WATER

1 CLOVE OF GARLIC, CRUSHED

1–2 SEABASS FILLETS
(AROUND 180G IN TOTAL)

SEA SALT AND FRESHLY
GROUND BLACK PEPPER

2 TSP COCONUT OIL

½ A RED ONION,
FINELY CHOPPED

6 STALKS OF ASPARAGUS,
HALVED

60G GREEN BEANS

½ A YELLOW PEPPER, SLICED

GROUND TURMERIC

CHILLI FLAKES

40G GREEN CABBAGE,
WASHED AND CUT INTO
FINGER-LENGTH PIECES

1 Rinse the rice, then drain and place in a pan. Pour over the water and bring to the boil. Lower the heat to a simmer, cover the pan and cook according to the packet instructions (these can vary), then drain.

2 Spread the crushed garlic on top of the seabass fillets (not the skin side). Season with salt and pepper.

3 Put 1 teaspoon of coconut oil into a frying pan and place on a medium heat. When the oil is hot, add the seabass to the pan, skin side down. Cook until crisp, then turn. It should take about 8 minutes in total.

4 Put another teaspoon of coconut oil into another pan on a medium heat, and when hot, add the red onion, asparagus, green beans, yellow pepper, and turmeric and chilli flakes to your taste. Stir for 2 minutes, then add the cabbage and the cooked rice. Cook, stirring gently, until heated through.

5 Serve the seabass on top of the rice and rainbow vegetables.

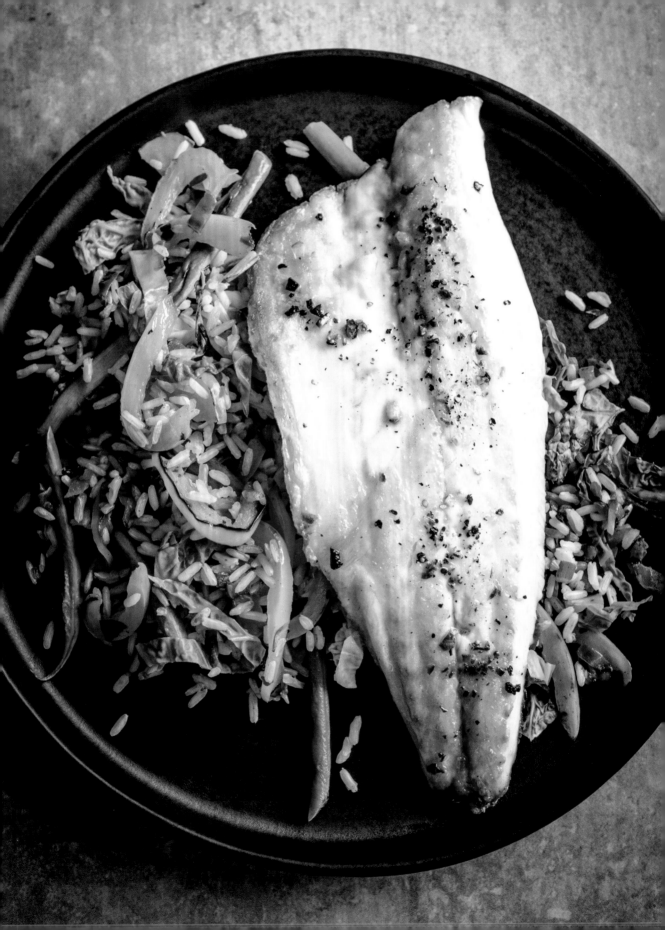

CURRIED LAMB WITH BANANA

Yes, I know: banana with lamb?! All I can say is, don't knock it until you've tried it. Opposites often attract, and this can apply to flavours too. In this instance, it's the sweetness of the mango chutney and the banana coupled with the savoury flavour of the curry that makes this so delicious. You'll see. I love brown rice with lamb. And generally if I like something, that tends to be it. If it ain't broke, don't fix it! But of course, you could serve it with any other grain or carb (see pages 224–9).

SERVES 2–3

500G LAMB (LEG OR SHOULDER WORK WELL, BUT YOU CAN USE ANY CUT)

A GOOD DRIZZLE OF COLD-PRESSED RAPESEED OIL

120G SWEET MANGO CHUTNEY

3 CLOVES OF GARLIC, CHOPPED

100ML DAIRY-FREE CREAM, SUCH AS SOYA

1–2 TSP CURRY POWDER

1 BANANA, SLICED

1 Preheat the oven to 180°C/160°C fan/gas 4.

2 Cut the lamb into chunks and place in a high-sided roasting tray. Drizzle with rapeseed oil, turning the lamb pieces so that they are all glazed. Roast for 20 minutes.

3 Put the chutney, garlic, cream and curry powder into a pan on a medium heat. Stir together and heat for a few minutes until hot, without letting it boil.

4 Remove the lamb from the oven and pour over the hot creamy mixture, then return to the oven for another 5 minutes. The sauce should be similar to yoghurt in consistency.

5 Serve topped with the sliced banana.

TERIYAKI MEATBALLS WITH MUSHROOMS

Whenever I eat this dish it fills my heart, as it reminds me of my home in Iceland. These meatballs are something my mum always makes when me and all my siblings are over for dinner. It's creamy, rich and so tasty. My mum really knows what she is doing. I've included a recipe for sweet potato mash, but these meatballs are also great served with noodles, brown rice or barley for soaking up the delicious sauce.

SERVES 3–4

FOR THE MEATBALLS

750G MINCED BEEF

200ML TERIYAKI SAUCE

1 TSP GROUND GINGER

1 TSP GARLIC POWDER

2 EGGS

1 TSP COCONUT OIL

1 X 290G TIN OF SLICED BUTTON MUSHROOMS

250G DAIRY-FREE CREAM, SUCH AS SOYA

SEA SALT AND FRESHLY GROUND BLACK PEPPER

FOR THE SWEET POTATO MASH

500G SWEET POTATOES (PARSNIPS OR CELERIAC WORK WELL TOO), PEELED AND CHOPPED

1 TSP VEGAN, GOAT'S OR SHEEP'S BUTTER, PLUS MORE TO TASTE

1 TSP GROUND NUTMEG, PLUS MORE TO TASTE

1 Preheat the oven to 180°C/160°C fan/gas 4.

2 In a large bowl mix together the beef, teriyaki sauce, ginger, garlic and eggs. Shape the mixture into large golfball-size balls.

3 Put the coconut oil into a casserole or ovenproof pan for which you have a lid, and place on a medium heat. When hot, fry the meatballs, turning to brown them on all sides – this will take a few minutes.

4 Pour over the mushrooms and their liquid and the cream, and season with salt and pepper. Put the lid on the pan, place in the oven and cook for 20 minutes.

5 To make the sweet potato mash, put the potatoes into a pan and add enough water to cover them and a pinch of salt if you like. Simmer until soft (stick a knife in to check if you're not sure – when it slides through, it's ready).

6 Remove from the heat and mash immediately, adding the butter and seasoning with the salt, pepper and the nutmeg as you mash. It won't be completely smooth but should have a good creamy texture. Taste and add more salt, pepper and nutmeg if you want.

PARSNIP & SWEET POTATO SOUP

Earthy, creamy parsnips and sweet potatoes make a hearty soup that's high in fibre, manganese and vitamin C.

SERVES 4

500G PARSNIPS, PEELED AND CHOPPED

500G SWEET POTATOES, PEELED AND CHOPPED

1 VEGETABLE STOCK CUBE, CRUMBLED

1 TSP GROUND NUTMEG

2 CLOVES OF GARLIC, CHOPPED

200ML DAIRY-FREE CREAM, SUCH AS SOYA

SEA SALT AND FRESHLY GROUND BLACK PEPPER

4 TSP OAT CREAM

A SPRINKLING OF CHOPPED FRESH PARSLEY

1 Put the parsnips and sweet potatoes into a pan and add enough water to cover. Place on a medium heat, bring to the boil, then simmer until soft (stick a knife in to check if you're not sure – when it slides through, it's ready).

2 Add the stock cube, nutmeg, garlic and dairy-free cream and mix together well. Season with salt and pepper.

3 Take off the heat and blend until smooth, using a hand-held electric blender.

4 To serve, ladle into bowls, adding a teaspoon of oat cream and a sprinkling of parsley to each bowl.

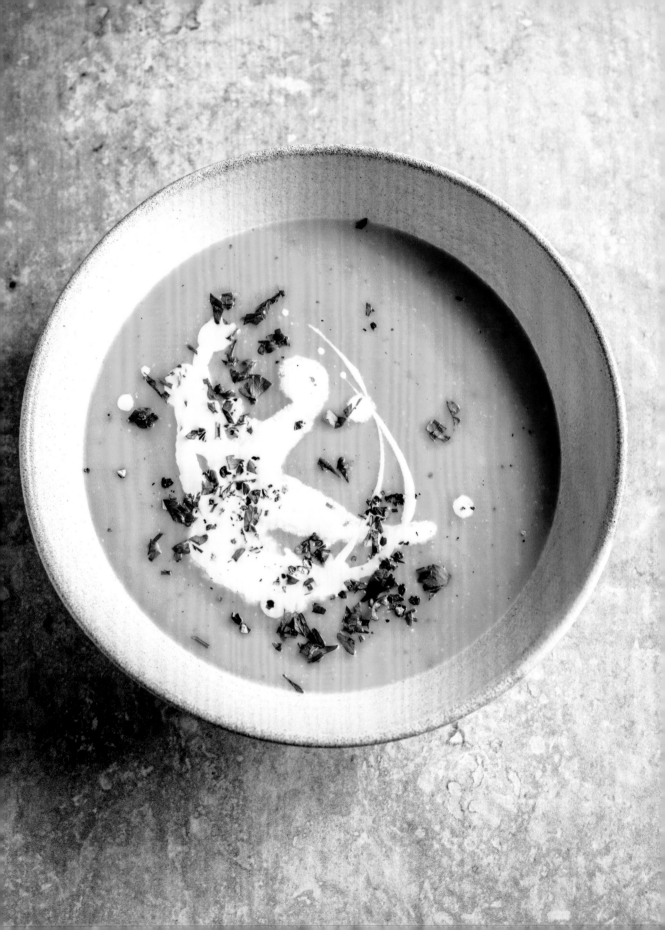

CARROT & COCONUT MILK SOUP

This soup has it all: spice, sweetness, and a slight sourness. Perfect served with a slice of Tyr's Post-war Treat (see page 151).

SERVES 4

1KG CARROTS, PEELED AND CHOPPED

1 ONION, FINELY CHOPPED

1 TSP GROUND CUMIN

1 TSP CURRY POWDER

A THUMB-SIZE PIECE OF GINGER, PEELED AND FINELY CHOPPED

1 CLOVE OF GARLIC

1 VEGETABLE STOCK CUBE, FINELY CHOPPED

1 X 400ML TIN OF COCONUT MILK

1 Put the carrots and onions into a pan with enough water to cover. Bring to the boil on a medium heat, then simmer until soft (stick a knife in to check if you're not sure – when it slides through, it's ready).

2 Stir in all the other ingredients, simmer for another 10 minutes, then remove from the heat.

3 Blend until smooth, using a hand-held electric blender.

TYR'S POST-WAR TREAT

Tyr is the god of war as well as the lawgiver. He is brave, powerful and gutsy, and this seedy rough-textured brown bread, filled with great energy, vitamins and minerals, is definitely what he would treat himself to after going berserk. It's so simple: you just mix it together, put it into the oven, and skál for you!

SERVES 1

500G OAT OR SPELT FLOUR

100G MIXED SEEDS (SESAME, SUNFLOWER AND PUMPKIN), PLUS EXTRA TO SPRINKLE ON TOP

½ TSP FINE SALT

3 TSP GLUTEN-FREE, ALUMINIUM-FREE BAKING POWDER

200ML RICE MILK

150ML BOILING WATER

1 Preheat the oven to 200°C/180°C fan/gas 6.

2 Put the flour, seeds, salt and baking powder into a large bowl and mix together.

3 Pour the rice milk into the boiling water and stir to combine.

4 Make a well in the flour mixture and slowly pour in the hot liquid, stirring slowly with a wooden spoon to bring it together. When it reaches an even, smooth, dough-like consistency, scrape it into a 900g non-stick loaf tin, sprinkling an extra handful of seeds on top.

5 Bake for 30 minutes, then take out of the tin and leave on a wire rack to cool.

IT'S A WRAP

Wraps are so simple, and are great for a speedy post-training lunch or dinner. You can chuck pretty much whatever's about into them, making them perfect for using up leftovers or any odds and ends in the fridge. You should feel free to riff on the following recipes: use them as guidelines and add or swap in what you already have. I often like to add a drizzle of goat's yoghurt to my wraps, but see the Sauces section (pages 212–5) for more ideas. Each wrap recipe serves 1.

VEGGIE HUMMUS WRAP

Eating healthily doesn't have to be complicated. This gorgeous wrap is full of crunch and takes hardly any time to put together.

SERVES 1

2 TBSP HUMMUS
(ORGANIC, IF POSSIBLE)

2 WHOLEWHEAT TORTILLA
WRAPS

50G KALE, FINELY CHOPPED

½ A SMALL CUCUMBER,
CUT INTO THIN MATCHSTICKS

½ AN AVOCADO, SLICED

¼ OF A RAW BEETROOT,
PEELED INTO THIN STRIPS

2 TSP SUNFLOWER SEEDS
(YOU CAN LIGHTLY TOAST THEM
IN A DRY PAN IF YOU LIKE)

A SMALL HANDFUL OF
FRESH BASIL LEAVES

SEA SALT AND FRESHLY
GROUND BLACK PEPPER

1 Spread a tablespoon of hummus over each of the two wraps.

2 Add the finely chopped kale, cucumber, avocado and beetroot. Top with the sunflower seeds and basil leaves and season with salt and pepper. Fold and enjoy!

TIP: Beetroot juice can go everywhere and tends to stain. So remember to wear an apron and wash your hands as soon as you've finished prepping.

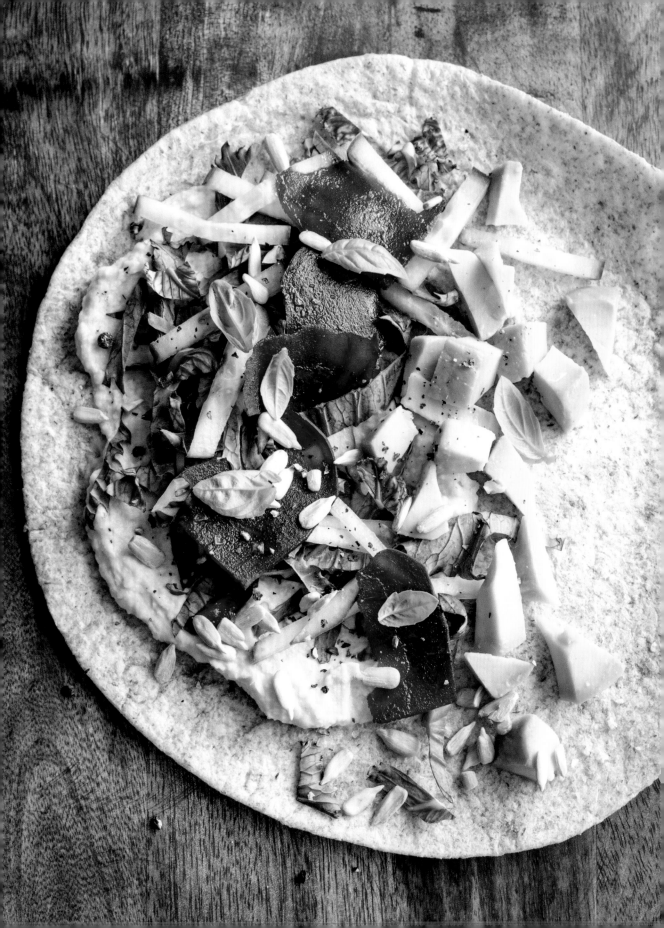

CHICKEN AND KIDNEY BEAN WRAP

Chicken: check. Greens: check. Avocado: check. Feta: check. All my favourite ingredients, wrapped up in one super quick meal.

SERVES 1

1 TSP COCONUT OIL

1 CHICKEN BREAST, CUT INTO BITE-SIZE PIECES

SEA SALT AND FRESHLY GROUND BLACK PEPPER

150G TINNED KIDNEY BEANS, DRAINED

3 BROCCOLI FLORETS

A HANDFUL OF KALE

50G GOAT'S MILK FETA

2 SMALL WHOLEWHEAT TORTILLA WRAPS

½ AN AVOCADO, SLICED

1 Preheat the oven to 180°C/160°C fan/gas 4.

2 Put the coconut oil into a pan and place on a medium heat. When hot, add the chicken and season with salt and pepper. Cook, stirring, until golden and cooked through – about 7–10 minutes.

3 Lay half the chicken, kidney beans, broccoli, kale and feta in the middle of each wrap, then fold and place in the oven for 10 minutes to warm through.

4 When the feta is slightly melted and everything is warm, remove the wraps from the oven and open a little, sliding the avocado in. Refold and enjoy.

ALL-DAY BREAKFAST WRAP

Who says breakfast is limited to the mornings? Being a Viking is all about living outside the box, which means this breakfast wrap is appropriate at any time of day . . . as long as you've trained!

SERVES 1

2 MEDIUM EGGS

1 CLOVE OF GARLIC, CHOPPED

A FEW FRESH CHIVES, CHOPPED

SEA SALT AND FRESHLY GROUND BLACK PEPPER

120G TINNED BORLOTTI BEANS, DRAINED

A DRIZZLE OF COLD-PRESSED RAPESEED OIL

4 RASHERS OF SMOKED STREAKY BACON

2 SMALL WHOLEWHEAT TORTILLA WRAPS

A SPLASH OF TABASCO SAUCE (OPTIONAL)

1 Crack the eggs into a medium bowl and whisk together. Mix in the garlic and chives and season with salt and pepper. Set aside.

2 Put the beans into a pan and place on a low heat, stirring and cooking for a few minutes. They are already cooked – you just want to heat them up.

3 Put the rapeseed oil into another pan and place on a medium-high heat. When the oil has melted and the pan is hot, put in the bacon and cook on each side until crispy.

4 Lower the heat to medium, then push the bacon to the side of the pan and add the garlicky eggs to the other side, stirring with a wooden spoon to scramble them into large curds. Right before you take everything out of the pan you can place the wraps on top for 30 seconds, just to warm them.

5 Spoon half the beans, scrambled eggs and bacon (you might want to break this up into bite-size pieces) into the middle of each wrap, adding a splash of Tabasco if you like. Fold and enjoy.

VEGGIE OPTION: Use 100g of halloumi instead of the bacon. Preheat the oven to 180°C/160°C fan/gas 4 and grease a small roasting tray with coconut oil. Cut the halloumi into 4 slices and place in the tray. Surround them with 6 halved cherry tomatoes. Season with salt and pepper and put into the oven for about 10–15 minutes (turning the halloumi once), or until the cheese has just begun to colour and the tomatoes have softened.

CHILLI BEEF WRAPS

Iron is an essential part of your diet, contributing to the transport of oxygen by your red blood cells and the transmission of nerve impulses, among other things. The beef and my favourite kidney beans in this substantial wrap are packed full of it. Perfect training day fuel.

SERVES 1

1 TSP COCONUT OIL

½ AN ONION, FINELY CHOPPED

1 CLOVE OF GARLIC, FINELY CHOPPED

150G MINCED BEEF

½ A BEEF STOCK CUBE, MIXED WITH 120ML BOILING WATER

1 TSP CHILLI POWDER

150G TINNED KIDNEY BEANS, DRAINED

3 LARGE BROCCOLI FLORETS

SEA SALT AND FRESHLY GROUND BLACK PEPPER

2 SMALL WHOLEWHEAT TORTILLA WRAPS

½ AN AVOCADO

1 Put the coconut oil into a pan and place on a medium heat. Once the pan is hot and the oil has melted, add the onion and garlic. Cook for 5 minutes, stirring occasionally, until softened and golden.

2 Add the minced beef and cook until browned and all the juice has evaporated (browning the meat really makes all the difference). Pour in the beef stock, then add the chilli powder and stir together. Cook for a couple more minutes.

3 Add the kidney beans and cook for 3 minutes, then add the broccoli for another 2 minutes. Cook until the kidney beans are heated through. Season with salt and pepper.

4 Right before you take everything out of the pan you can place the wraps on top for 30 seconds, just to warm them.

5 Peel and slice the avocado, and place half in the middle of each wrap, spooning the mince mixture on top. Fold and enjoy.

TUNA & HALLOUMI MELT WRAP

Packed with omega-3s, protein, vitamin C, vitamin B12 and many more vitamins and minerals, tuna is part of the strong Viking food clan! This is a delicious wrap: the cooked dates are so sweet and go perfectly with the halloumi and the other ingredients.

SERVES 1

1 X 160G TIN OF TUNA, DRAINED

6 DATES, PITTED AND CHOPPED

4 SPRING ONIONS, FINELY SLICED

3 BROCCOLI FLORETS, FINELY CHOPPED

½ A RED ONION, FINELY CHOPPED

SEA SALT AND FRESHLY GROUND BLACK PEPPER

2 WHOLEWHEAT TORTILLA WRAPS

100G HALLOUMI, CUT INTO 6–8 SLICES

A FEW LEAVES OF LITTLE GEM OR OTHER LETTUCE, FINELY SLICED

A DRIZZLE OF SALSA (SEE PAGE 215)

1 Preheat the oven to 200°C/180°C fan/gas 6.

2 In a small bowl, mix together the tuna, dates, spring onions, broccoli and red onion and season with salt and pepper to taste.

3 Place half the tuna mix on one half of each wrap and cover with the halloumi slices. Fold the other half of each wrap over and put on a baking tray. Put into the oven for about 7–10 minutes, then remove, open each wrap and add the lettuce along with a drizzle of salsa. Refold and enjoy.

VEGGIE OPTION: Replace the tuna with 150g of tinned butter beans or chickpeas, slightly mashing them before mixing them with the other ingredients.

ANYTIME MEALS

Anytime Meals are for when you haven't trained before eating. They are high in protein and healthy fats, with your carb intake coming from vegetables and fibrous fruits, the Always Carbs (see page 11). The recipes in the Anytime Meals section can be eaten for lunch and dinner on rest days. They should also be eaten on training days when you haven't yet trained. For example, if you are training after lunch, you would eat an Anytime Meal for lunch. With all the Anytime recipes, you can always add a portion of Sometimes Carbs (see pages 224–9) and make it a Post-training Meal when your body needs more energy. I have made suggestions for what might work well throughout, but of course you can choose whatever you like.

All dishes serve one person, unless otherwise stated.

» OXIDATIVE STRESS

Oxidative stress is the disturbance in the balance between the production of free radicals (free radicals are unstable atoms that can damage cells, causing illness and ageing) and antioxidants (the substances that counteract them, warding off cell damage by removing the free radicals before they can do harm).

Take out/limit the things that create this stress: alcohol, fried and barbecued food, lack of sleep, very high-intensity training lasting more than an hour, constant eating and drinking.

Sugars/carbs create much more oxidative stress than fats and proteins. The more sugar we eat, the more oxidation (i.e. the more free radical production) happens. Also, sugar does not suppress ghrelin (the hunger hormone) and also does not stimulate leptin (the satiety hormone), meaning you are constantly hungry and over-eat, bringing a huge amount of free radical formation into the body. It's the worst cycle to create.

STEAMED COD AND FENNEL

Fennel is fantastic for a powerful Viking heart, as it's packed full of fibre, potassium, folate, and vitamins B6 and C, which all appear to support great heart health. Plus its sweet, aniseedy flavour goes so well with delicate white fish like cod. Serve with a salad of your choosing (see pages 206–11) – I like to add goat's cheese feta, as I think it goes perfectly with this dish!

SERVES 2

1 TBSP VEGAN, GOAT'S OR SHEEP'S BUTTER

A DRIZZLE OF COLD-PRESSED RAPESEED OIL

1 LARGE FENNEL BULB, TRIMMED AND FINELY SLICED

4 COD FILLETS, SKINLESS AND BONELESS

SEA SALT AND FRESHLY GROUND BLACK PEPPER

1 LEMON, HALVED

1 Put the butter and oil into a sauté pan for which you have a lid and place on a medium heat (the oil has a higher burning point than the butter, so stops it burning). When the butter is melted and the pan is hot, add the sliced fennel and cook, stirring, until softened – about 5 minutes.

2 Place the cod on top of the fennel, season with salt and pepper and lower the heat slightly. Cover with the lid and cook for 12 minutes, or until the fish is cooked (gently insert a knife to check if you're unsure: the fish should flake easily, and be white throughout).

3 Remove from the heat, and squeeze over the lemon juice before serving.

POST-TRAINING OPTION: The fluffy texture of quinoa pairs perfectly with this recipe (see page 228).

TANGY STIR-FRIED TOFU & VEGETABLES

My dear friend Saffron lives in India – she has lived in many different places in India but when she first moved there she lived for years in Rishikesh, where she managed an orphanage and a school. Saffron is one of the greats. There, she met and worked with people from all over the world, which is why her food is so diversely put together. And whenever she and her husband come to London they stay with me and my daughter, Raven. Thanks to them I have learned some extremely yummy combinations. Vikings love fusion, and this vegetarian stir-fry is a favourite.

SERVES 1

1 TBSP SESAME OIL

2 CLOVES OF GARLIC, FINELY CHOPPED

A THUMB-SIZE PIECE OF GINGER, GRATED

100G TOFU, CHOPPED INTO 1½CM CUBES

1 MEDIUM CARROT, FINELY SLICED INTO STRIPS

2 PORTOBELLO MUSHROOMS, ROUGHLY CHOPPED

1 PAK CHOI, ROUGHLY CHOPPED

3 TBSP SOY SAUCE

1 TSP RAW HONEY

70G SPINACH, WASHED

1 TSP SESAME SEEDS

1 Put the sesame oil into a wok (or a pan) on a medium to high heat. When the oil is hot (but not smoking), add the garlic and ginger, stir-fry for 10 seconds until fragrant, then add the tofu. Stir-fry for 2–3 minutes, until the tofu starts to turn golden brown.

2 Turn the heat down to medium and add the carrot, mushrooms, pak choi and soy sauce to the pan. Stir-fry for around 5 minutes, until the vegetables are tender.

3 Drizzle in the honey, mixing to incorporate, then add the spinach and stir-fry for 1 minute until it begins to wilt.

4 To toast the sesame seeds (this can be done in advance), simply place a small pan on a medium-low heat. Cook the seeds for a few minutes, stirring occasionally, until fragrant and just starting to colour. Sprinkle over the stir-fry.

POST-TRAINING OPTION: Rice or egg noodles make an excellent addition (see page 228 for cooking instructions). Add a splash more soy sauce and an extra drizzle of honey, if you like.

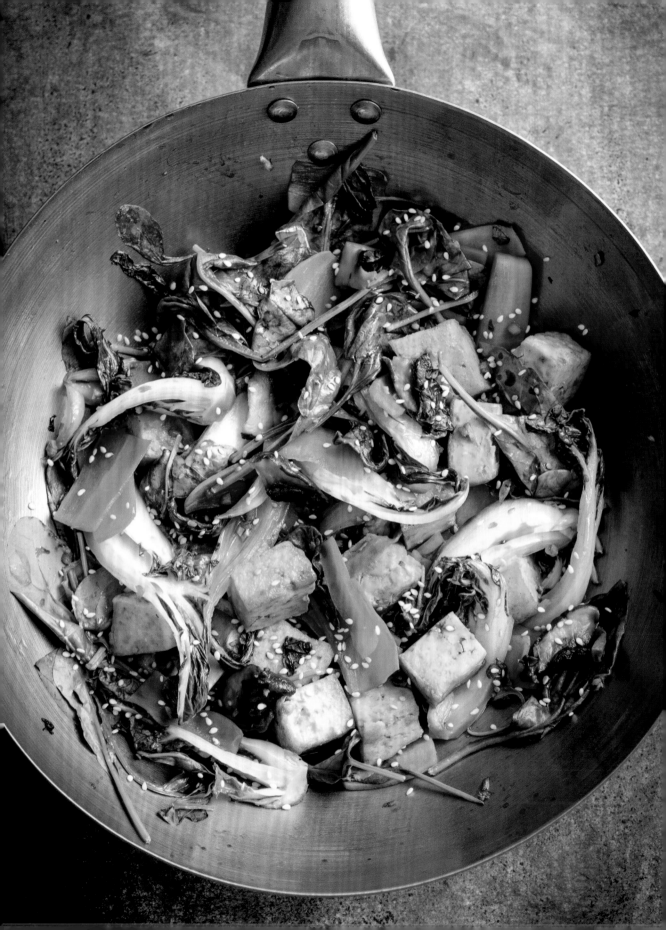

SEARED SEABASS WITH SPICY RED PEPPER SALSA

A meal with an energy-lifting kick. Cayenne pepper benefits your gut, and studies have suggested it may speed up your metabolism, aid your digestion and promote heart health. So why not add some quality spice to your life!

SERVES 1

1 TSP COCONUT OIL, OR COLD-PRESSED RAPESEED OIL

180G SEABASS FILLETS (1–2, DEPENDING ON SIZE)

SEA SALT AND FRESHLY GROUND BLACK PEPPER

½ A COURGETTE, CUT INTO CHUNKS

70G SPINACH, WASHED

1 RED PEPPER, DESEEDED AND FINELY SLICED

3 CHERRY TOMATOES, HALVED

¼ OF A RED ONION, FINELY CHOPPED

1 TBSP SALSA (SEE PAGE 215)

1 TSP CAYENNE PEPPER

A HANDFUL OF FRESH BASIL, LEAVES AND STALKS, FINELY CHOPPED

1 Put the oil into a pan and place on a medium heat. When hot, season the seabass with salt and pepper and add to the pan, skin side down. Cook for about 6 minutes, turning once, then remove from the pan.

2 Add the courgettes and spinach to the pan and cook for 2–3 minutes.

3 In a medium bowl, mix the red pepper, cherry tomatoes and onion with the salsa, cayenne pepper and basil.

4 Transfer the seabass, spinach and courgettes to a plate and spoon the salsa mixture on top of the fish before serving.

POST-TRAINING OPTION: Mix some nutty barley (see page 228) in with the red pepper salsa.

CAJUN-SPICED CHICKEN WITH HALLOUMI

Who can resist grilled halloumi? I know I can't! Especially when it's combined with soft shallots and tangy spices, as here.

SERVES 1

1 LARGE CHICKEN BREAST, CHOPPED INTO BITE-SIZE PIECES

1½ TSP CAJUN SPICE

½ TSP PAPRIKA

1 TSP COCONUT OIL, OR COLD-PRESSED RAPESEED OIL

½ A SHALLOT, FINELY CHOPPED

80G HALLOUMI, CHOPPED INTO 1CM CHUNKS

6 CLOSED-CUP MUSHROOMS, ROUGHLY CHOPPED

4 CAULIFLOWER FLORETS, ROUGHLY CHOPPED

70G SPINACH, WASHED

SEA SALT AND FRESHLY GROUND BLACK PEPPER

1 A couple of hours before you want to cook, put the chicken into a small bowl with the spices, mix together, then cover and pop into the fridge to marinate.

2 Put the oil into a pan and place on a medium-high heat. When hot, add the marinated chicken and cook for 7–10 minutes, turning halfway through, until it's crisp and golden brown on the outside and white and juicy inside. Remove the chicken from the pan.

3 Lower the heat to medium and add the shallots and halloumi to the pan. Cook for a few minutes, stirring the shallots until they have softened, and turning the halloumi until it's golden all over.

4 Remove the halloumi from the pan, then add the mushrooms and cauliflower and continue to cook (blanch the cauliflower beforehand if you prefer it softer: bring a small pan of water to the boil and cook the cauliflower for couple of minutes before removing with a slotted spoon). Once the mushrooms are tender, add the spinach and cook until it starts to wilt.

5 Season the vegetables with salt and pepper and serve with the halloumi, alongside the chicken.

POST-TRAINING OPTION: Add 150g of tinned butter beans: just add them to the pan at the same time as the mushrooms and stir to warm through.

VEGGIE OPTION: Remove the chicken and instead add some organic firm tofu. Cut the tofu into 1cm cubes, then cook in the same way as the chicken, marinating and frying for 7–10 minutes.

ROASTED TUNA STEAK & MIXED VEGETABLES

A juicy, colourful recipe that is done in the blink of an eye – and using just one tray, too. This is great after a long day when you can't be bothered to spend too long in the kitchen but still want something tasty and nutritious.

SERVES 1

1 CARROT, CHOPPED INTO BATONS

½ A SMALL COURGETTE, SLICED

3 CHERRY TOMATOES, HALVED

½ A RED PEPPER, DESEEDED AND SLICED

1 CLOVE OF GARLIC, FINELY CHOPPED

1 TSP COLD-PRESSED RAPESEED OIL

SEA SALT AND FRESHLY GROUND BLACK PEPPER

1 TUNA STEAK (APPROX. 150G)

JUICE FROM ½ A LEMON

50G KALE

4 BROCCOLI FLORETS

GARLIC SALT

1 Preheat the oven to 200°C/180°C fan/gas 6 and line a roasting tray with foil.

2 Place the carrots, courgettes, tomatoes and red peppers in the roasting tray and sprinkle over the garlic. Drizzle with the oil and season with salt and pepper, then mix together with your hands. Put into the oven for around 7 minutes, until the vegetables are starting to colour.

3 Add the tuna to the tray, season with salt and pepper and squeeze over the lemon juice. Return to the oven for around 4 minutes, then turn the tuna over and roast for a final 4 minutes. For those final minutes, throw in the kale and broccoli. The tuna should have lost all of its pinkness on the outside when it is ready.

4 Season with garlic salt before serving.

POST-TRAINING OPTION: Add 150g of tinned chickpeas. Add them to the tray first, drizzling with the oil, then put into the oven and cook for 20 minutes. Then, as above, add the vegetables apart from the kale and broccoli. Cook for 7 minutes. Add the tuna with a squeeze of lemon juice for 4 minutes, turn it over, then throw in the kale and broccoli for the final 4 minutes.

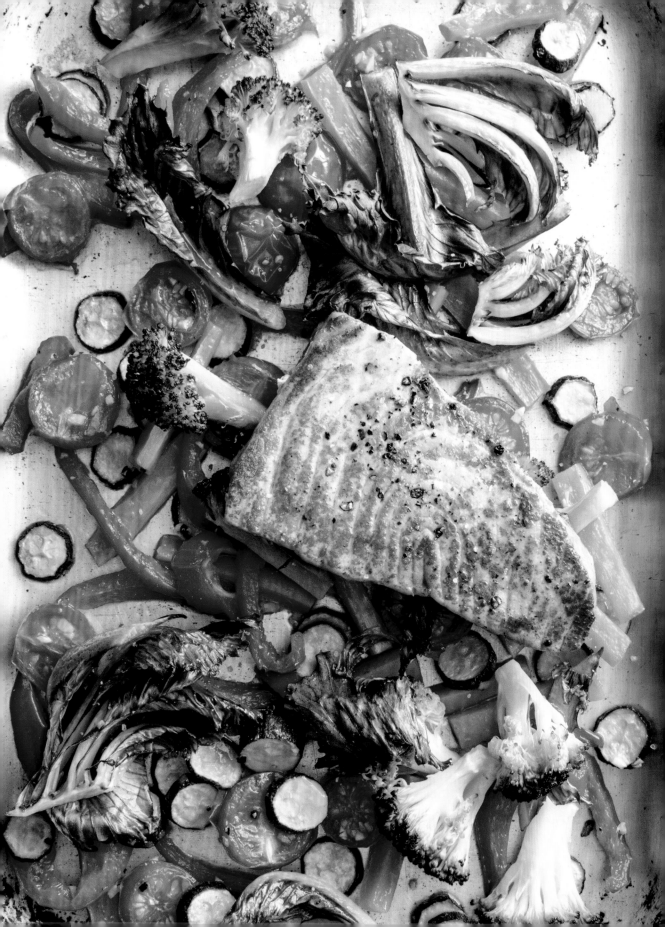

CHICKEN & GOLDEN CAULIFLOWER RICE

Crunchy, filling and packed with vitamin C, cauliflower rice tastes fantastic and is an easy way of adding more veg to your diet. The turmeric and curry powder make it really flavourful and satisfying, turning the cauliflower pieces a brilliant vibrant yellow. A meal to make you go for gold!

SERVES 1

1 WHOLE CAULIFLOWER, TRIMMED AND ROUGHLY CHOPPED

1 TSP COCONUT OIL

1 TSP GROUND TURMERIC

1 TSP MEDIUM CURRY POWDER

SEA SALT

½ A RED PEPPER, DESEEDED AND CHOPPED

5 SPRING ONIONS, CHOPPED

3 CHERRY TOMATOES, HALVED

1 LARGE COOKED CHICKEN BREAST

½ AN AVOCADO, SLICED

A SPOONFUL OF SHEEP'S MILK YOGHURT (OPTIONAL)

1 Preheat the oven to 180°C/160°C fan/gas 4.

2 Roughly chop the cauliflower, then blitz it to small pieces in a food processor – it should look similar to quinoa.

3 Spread the coconut oil on a baking tray. Add the cauliflower, turmeric, curry powder and a pinch of salt, and mix together so that the cauliflower is evenly coated with the spices. Mix in the red pepper, spring onions and cherry tomatoes, making sure all the ingredients are evenly distributed. Roast for 20 minutes, until tender.

4 Serve the cauliflower rice with the chicken, the sliced avocado and a drizzle of yoghurt.

POST-TRAINING OPTION: 15 minutes into the cooking time, mix 150g of cooked kidney beans or chickpeas through the cauliflower rice and veg and pop back into the oven for the last 5 minutes.

VEGGIE OPTION: Black beans fit extremely well with the flavour and texture of the cauliflower rice and spices. Go to Sometimes Carbs (page 224) for instructions. Halloumi (120g, cut in slices and cooked on a griddle pan, 4 minutes on each side or until golden) is also extremely delicious with the cauliflower rice. Your choice!

ROASTED VEGETABLES WITH FETA & SEEDS

This is one of those recipes that is so much more than the sum of its parts in terms of flavour and satisfaction. They may be small, but seeds are Viking mainstays in terms of nutrition: a great source of protein and unsaturated fats, and packed full of vitamins.

SERVES 2

1 COURGETTE, ROUGHLY CHOPPED

1 RED PEPPER, DESEEDED AND ROUGHLY CHOPPED

1 SMALL RED ONION, ROUGHLY CHOPPED

2 TBSP COLD-PRESSED RAPESEED OIL

SEA SALT AND FRESHLY GROUND BLACK PEPPER

100G GOAT'S MILK FETA

FOR THE SEEDS

25G SUNFLOWER SEEDS

25G PUMPKIN SEEDS

15G SESAME SEEDS

1 TBSP DARK SOY SAUCE

½ TBSP COLD-PRESSED RAPESEED OIL

1 Preheat the oven to 200°C/180°C fan/gas 6.

2 Spread the chopped veg on a baking tray, drizzle with oil and season well with salt and pepper. Roast for 20 minutes, giving everything a shuffle halfway through to help it cook evenly.

3 While the veg are in the oven, roast the seeds. Place all the seeds on a baking tray, drizzle over the soy sauce and oil, then mix together with your hands, making sure they're well coated. Roast for 7–8 minutes, stirring with a wooden spoon every 2 or 3 minutes, until the seeds are lightly coloured and the pumpkin seeds have puffed up. Remove from the oven and leave to cool slightly.

4 A couple of minutes before the veg are cooked, crumble over the feta and put back into the oven to melt slightly. Sprinkle over the seeds before serving.

POST-TRAINING OPTION: This works really well with fluffy quinoa (see page 228), or spooned over a slice of toast.

SALSA CHICKEN

This recipe is a great reason to make salsa (see page 215). Spring onions are such a versatile ingredient and are easy to use up when cooking meals for one or two, as you're never left with half an onion in the fridge! I also like using them because research suggests that they are fantastic for cardiovascular health, can reduce blood pressure and cholesterol, boost the immune system and speed up blood circulation.

SERVES 1

1 LARGE BONELESS SKINLESS CHICKEN BREAST

1 HEAPED TSP DIJON MUSTARD

SEA SALT AND FRESHLY GROUND BLACK PEPPER

1 TSP COCONUT OIL, OR COLD-PRESSED RAPESEED OIL

3–4 TBSP SALSA (SEE PAGE 215), MIXED WITH THE JUICE OF 1 LIME

3 SPRING ONIONS, CHOPPED

2 LARGE BROCCOLI FLORETS, CHOPPED

½ AN AVOCADO, SLICED

8 ALMONDS, CHOPPED VERY FINELY

1 Coat the chicken breast with the mustard and season with salt and pepper.

2 Put the oil into a large pan and place on a high heat. When hot, add the chicken and cook for 4 minutes. Turn it over, reduce the heat to medium, then spoon over the salsa-lime mixture and add the spring onions.

3 Simmer, uncovered, for around 8–10 minutes, until the chicken is completely cooked through (cut into it to check, if unsure) and the sauce has thickened.

4 Remove the chicken to a plate. Turn the heat back up to high and continue to cook the sauce for about 30 seconds, then add the broccoli for a minute or two, until just tender (I like my broccoli on the crunchier side, but you can cook it a bit longer if you prefer it softer).

5 Pour the sauce over the chicken and top with sliced avocado and chopped almonds.

POST-TRAINING OPTION: I like to add brown rice with a teaspoon of curry powder mixed through it.

ICELANDIC-INSPIRED POACHED COD

Cod always reminds me of Iceland and being little. It's funny – then I would be like, 'God, not fish again,' whereas now I say to my daughter, 'Let's have fish, Raven!' I have turned into my mother. This is how I like to poach cod, served alongside some of my favourite ingredients.

SERVES 1

1 TSP COCONUT OIL, OR COLD-PRESSED RAPESEED OIL

60G HALLOUMI, CUT INTO 1CM CUBES

6 CLOSED-CUP MUSHROOMS, SLICED

SEA SALT AND FRESHLY GROUND BLACK PEPPER

70G SPINACH, WASHED

400ML ALMOND MILK

½ A RED ONION, THINLY SLICED

1 CLOVE OF GARLIC, CHOPPED

1 DRIED BAY LEAF, FINELY CHOPPED

1 FRESH BAY LEAF

A FEW SPRIGS OF FRESH THYME

2 SMALL COD FILLETS

½ AN AVOCADO, SLICED

1 Preheat the oven to 200°C/180°C fan/gas 6.

2 Spread the coconut oil on a baking tray (or drizzle with rapeseed oil, if using), add the halloumi and mushrooms, and season with salt and pepper. Place in the oven and cook for 10–15 minutes, until soft and golden, adding the spinach to the tray for the last minute.

3 Pour the milk into a pan and add the onion, garlic, both bay leaves and the thyme. Place on a medium heat and bring to the boil, stirring continuously, then reduce the heat to a simmer.

4 Add the cod to the infused milk and continue to simmer for 7–8 minutes.

5 Carefully lift the cod out of the pan and on to a plate, then scoop out the onion, garlic and thyme, discarding the bay leaf (a slotted spoon is handy here), and place on top of the fish. Serve with the baked halloumi, mushrooms and spinach, and with the sliced avocado alongside.

POST-TRAINING OPTION: Add sweet potato fries (see Sometimes Carbs, page 227) for Viking-style fish and chips!

CAJUN GOAT'S MILK YOGHURT CHICKEN

The longer you marinate chicken, the more flavoursome and tender it becomes. A few hours in the fridge will make it extremely juicy, so it's worth prepping ahead if you have the time.

SERVES 1

1 LARGE CHICKEN BREAST, DICED

200ML GOAT'S MILK YOGHURT

2 TSP CAJUN SPICE

1 TSP PAPRIKA

1 TSP COCONUT OIL

A SMALL THUMB-SIZE PIECE OF GINGER, GRATED

1 CLOVE OF GARLIC, CHOPPED

½ A RED PEPPER, DESEEDED AND CHOPPED

4 SPRING ONIONS, CHOPPED

½ A CHICKEN STOCK CUBE, CRUMBLED

4 BROCCOLI FLORETS

70G SPINACH, WASHED

SEA SALT AND FRESHLY GROUND BLACK PEPPER

1 Put the chicken into a medium-size bowl with the yoghurt, Cajun spice and paprika, and mix together well. Cover with clingfilm and pop into the fridge for at least half an hour, and ideally a couple of hours.

2 Put the oil into a pan and place on a medium heat. When hot, add the ginger and garlic and stir-fry for a minute, until fragrant. Add the red pepper and spring onions and sauté, stirring, for a minute.

3 Using a spatula, add the chicken and all its yoghurt marinade to the pan, along with the stock cube. Stir to combine, then simmer gently until the chicken is cooked through – about 8 minutes. (If you're unsure, cut into a piece to check.)

4 When the chicken is cooked, add the broccoli and spinach to the pan for a minute and season with salt and pepper. The broccoli should be cooked but with a bite to it, and the spinach wilted (I like my broccoli on the crunchier side, but you can cook it a bit longer if you prefer it softer).

5 Plate up and enjoy, Viking!

POST-TRAINING OPTION: Add 100g of cooked barley (see page 228), season with salt, pepper and a teaspoon of paprika, and mix together well.

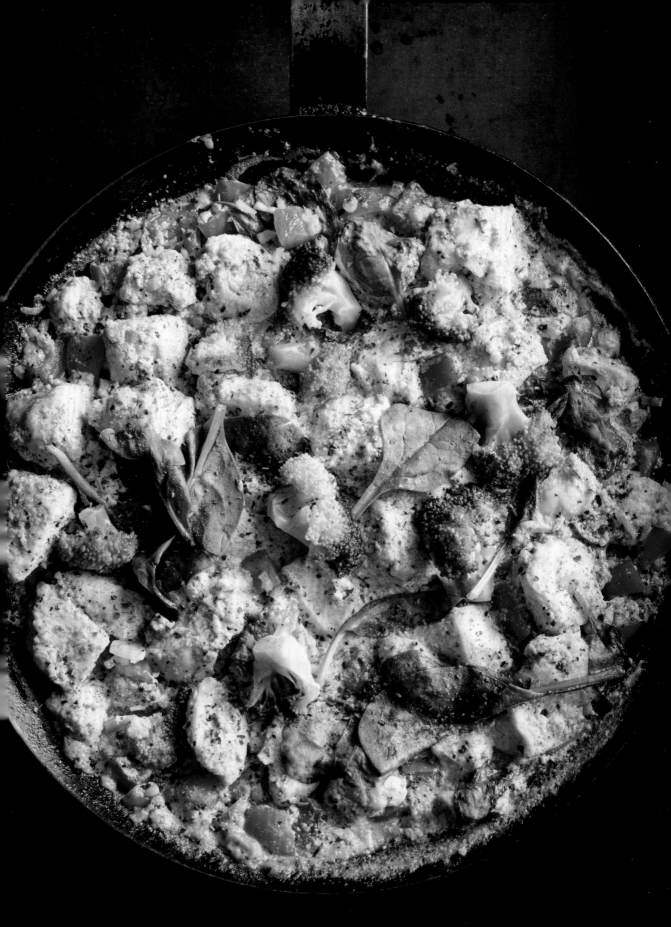

CHICKEN FAJITA SALAD

Everything that's delicious about chicken fajitas, just without the wraps. Rich in deliciousness and very rich in antioxidants and anti-inflammatories.

SERVES 1

½ AN AVOCADO, CHOPPED

1 TBSP SALSA (SEE PAGE 215)

2 CLOVES OF GARLIC, CHOPPED

1 TSP GROUND CUMIN

1 TSP DRIED OREGANO

1 TSP CHILLI POWDER

SEA SALT

1 LARGE CHICKEN BREAST, SLICED INTO LONG PIECES

1 TBSP COCONUT OIL, OR COLD-PRESSED RAPESEED OIL

½ A RED ONION, FINELY CHOPPED

1 SMALL RED PEPPER, DESEEDED AND SLICED

JUICE OF ½–1 LIME

1 LITTLE GEM LETTUCE, WASHED AND CHOPPED

JUICE OF 1 LEMON

1 Roughly mash the avocado in a small bowl and mix in the salsa.

2 Put the garlic, cumin, oregano, chilli powder and a pinch of salt into a medium bowl and mix together. Toss the chicken in the mixture until fully coated.

3 Put the oil into a large pan and place on a medium heat. When hot, sauté the onion for around 3 minutes, then add the chicken and cook for around 8–10 minutes, until it is golden brown and fully cooked through.

4 Add the red pepper to the pan with the lime juice – start with the juice of ½ a lime and add more if you think it needs it. Cook for 3 minutes, until the pepper has softened.

5 Serve the chicken with the lettuce and the avocado-salsa mix. Squeeze the lemon juice over to finalize the greatness!

POST-TRAINING OPTION: Add a couple of wholewheat tortilla wraps and wrap it up!

THOR-RED SALMON

Fish has always been a huge part of the Nordic diet and has sustained strong Vikings through the ages. An oily fish, salmon is bursting with nutrients and is an excellent source of vitamin B12, vitamin D, selenium, omega-3 fatty acids, phosphorus and vitamin B6, as well as a great source of protein. Food to keep you as fighting fit as the red-haired god of thunder.

SERVES 1

1 TBSP COCONUT OIL, OR COLD-PRESSED RAPESEED OIL

1–2 SALMON FILLETS (120G EACH)

2 TSP VEGAN RED PESTO (GLUTEN, DAIRY AND WHEAT FREE)

½ A COURGETTE, CHOPPED

3 CHERRY TOMATOES, HALVED

½ A RED PEPPER, DESEEDED AND CHOPPED

1 LARGE CLOVE OF GARLIC, CHOPPED

½ A RED ONION, SLICED

SEA SALT AND FRESHLY GROUND BLACK PEPPER

50G GOAT'S MILK FETA

1 Preheat the oven to 200°C/180°C fan/gas 6.

2 Line a roasting tray with foil and spread the coconut oil over it, or drizzle with the rapeseed oil. Place the salmon in the middle, and spoon the pesto on top, covering the fish evenly.

3 Scatter the courgettes, tomatoes, peppers, garlic and onions around the salmon, mixing everything together to combine, then season with salt and pepper and roast for 20 minutes. The vegetables should be golden when done, and the salmon an opaque, solid pink.

4 About 4 minutes before it's ready, dot the feta around the veg and put back into the oven until it's warmed through and starting to melt.

5 Transfer the salmon and vegetables with the gorgeous melted feta to a plate and enjoy.

POST-TRAINING OPTION: 100g of cooked nutty brown rice goes so well with the rich oily salmon.

SIRLOIN STEAK WITH FILLED PORTOBELLO MUSHROOMS

I am a sucker for a quality steak; I usually have red meat once or twice a week, and sirloin is my favourite! It's such a treat, and this recipe, full of rich, juicy flavour and texture, is something I always look forward to.

SERVES 1

2 PORTOBELLO MUSHROOMS

70G HALLOUMI

250G SIRLOIN STEAK, AROUND 3CM THICK

1 TSP COLD-PRESSED RAPESEED OIL

SEA SALT AND FRESHLY GROUND BLACK PEPPER

3 BROCCOLI FLORETS

70G SPINACH, WASHED

1 TBSP HUMMUS

1 Preheat the oven to 200°C/180°C fan/gas 6.

2 Cut off the mushroom stalk so you are left with two mushroom caps for stuffing.

3 Cut the halloumi into thin slices, then turn the mushrooms upside down and fill with the cheese. Place on a baking tray and roast in the oven for 10 minutes.

4 Rub the steak with the oil and season with salt and pepper on both sides. Put a frying pan on a medium-high heat. Put the steak into the pan. I like steak medium rare, so I cook it for 3–4 minutes on each side. Adjust the cooking time according to taste (around 2–3 minutes for rare, and 5–6 minutes for well done, depending on the thickness of your steak). When cooked to your liking, remove from the heat to a plate or board and leave to rest.

5 Boil enough water in a pan to cover the broccoli and spinach. Cook the veg for less than a minute, then drain.

6 Place the steak on a plate, with the mushrooms, the broccoli and spinach, and the hummus.

POST-TRAINING OPTION: Peel a medium sweet potato and cut it into 1cm rounds. Grill in a hot pan with a teaspoon of oil for 10 minutes, or until soft and caramelized. Season and serve with the steak.

TIP: Avoid overcooking the steak by pressing your finger into it gently after turning. You want it soft and juicy on the inside, therefore you should be able to press down into it easily. When it's browned but still has a bit of give, take it off the heat – remember it will continue to cook while it rests.

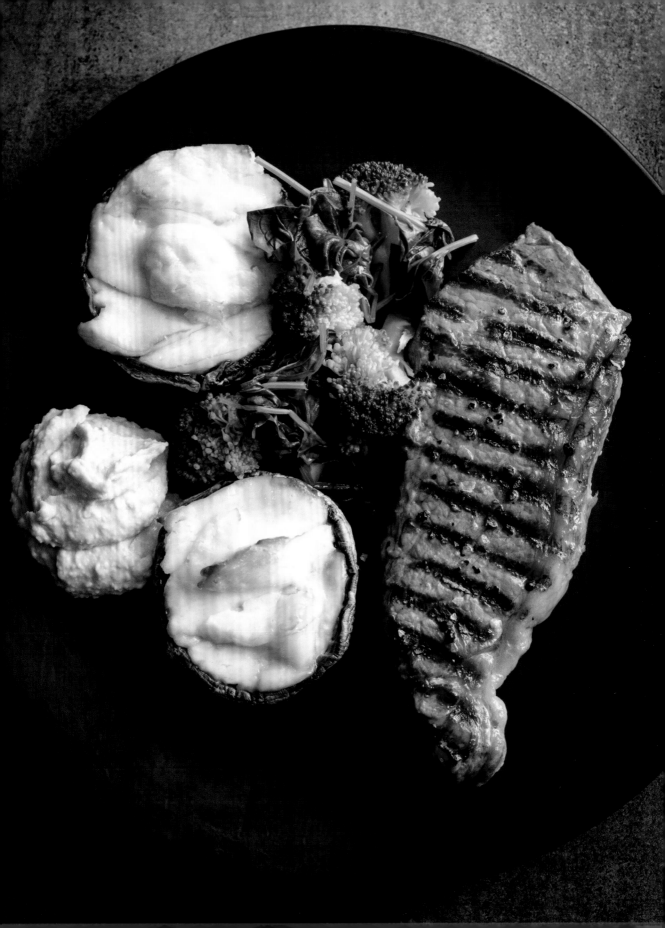

CHICKEN WITH WINE & BUTTERY MUSHROOMS

We Vikings love hygge, and with its buttery sauce this is comfort in a dish. The wine adds such a nice flavour to the chicken – it's well worth adding. Hygge is the word we Nordic people use for the warm, heart-filling enjoyments of life: a wonderful dinner by candlelight, reading all snuggled up on the sofa, enjoying cosy evenings with our loved ones. The little things that give us contentment and a feeling of peace and love.

SERVES 2

1 TSP COCONUT OIL

4 CHICKEN THIGHS, SKIN ON, BONE IN

SEA SALT AND FRESHLY GROUND BLACK PEPPER

½ AN ONION, FINELY CHOPPED

1 CLOVE OF GARLIC, FINELY CHOPPED

2 TBSP TOMATO PURÉE

2 SPRIGS OF FRESH THYME

3 SPRIGS OF FRESH PARSLEY, CHOPPED

50ML WHITE WINE

A KNOB OF GOAT'S BUTTER

100G CLOSED-CUP MUSHROOMS, CHOPPED

1 Preheat the oven to 200°C/180°C fan/gas 6.

2 Line a roasting tin (or a high-sided baking tray) with foil and spread over the coconut oil. Place the chicken thighs in the middle, season with salt and pepper, and roast for 10 minutes, until starting to brown.

3 Put the onion, garlic, tomato purée, thyme, parsley and wine into a pan and place on a medium heat. Simmer, stirring, for 5 minutes.

4 Remove the chicken from the oven and pour the hot aromatic liquid over it, then cover the roasting tin with foil and return it to the oven for 30 minutes.

5 While the chicken is cooking, put the butter into a pan on a medium heat. When melted, sauté the mushrooms for around 3–4 minutes or until golden brown and juicy, seasoning them with salt and pepper at the end.

6 Serve the chicken and its sauce in a soup plate or other high-rimmed plate, with the mushrooms alongside.

POST-TRAINING OPTION: Add 100g of cooked brown rice, mixing it with the mushrooms and their butter.

CHICKEN STIR-FRY WITH EDAMAME

Stir-frying is one of my favourite ways to cook vegetables – it's so quick and easy, and you still retain that vital crunch. Edamame are young green soya beans: they are a great plant-based form of protein and are high in the B vitamin folate, which helps to make red blood cells. If you can't find them fresh, they are readily available frozen.

SERVES 1

1 TSP COCONUT OIL

1 LARGE CHICKEN BREAST, CUT INTO BITE-SIZE CUBES

1 CLOVE OF GARLIC, CHOPPED

2 TSP GRATED GINGER

1 MEDIUM CARROT, CUT INTO BATONS

35G LEEKS, SLICED

50G MUSHROOMS, CHOPPED

2 TSP LIME JUICE

2 TBSP WARM WATER

SEA SALT

7 FRESH EDAMAME PODS

1–2 TBSP TERIYAKI SAUCE, ACCORDING TO TASTE

1 Put the coconut oil into a pan and place on a medium heat. When it's hot, add the chicken and stir-fry for around 8 minutes, until it's golden brown on the outside and cooked through on the inside.

2 Add the garlic and ginger to the pan and stir-fry for a minute, until fragrant. Add the carrots, leeks, mushrooms, lime juice and water. Stir-fry for a couple of minutes, until the carrots are cooked but with a slight bite to them.

3 Meanwhile, bring a pan of water to the boil with a pinch of salt. Add the edamame and cook for 4 minutes, then drain and sprinkle over a little salt.

4 Arrange the chicken and vegetable stir-fry on a plate, with the edamame on the side, and drizzle the teriyaki sauce over the top.

POST-TRAINING OPTION: Add a nest of egg noodles, which will go perfectly with this dish! Cook according to the packet instructions, drain, and add to the pan at the last minute, just to mix them in.

VEGGIE OPTION: Use 100g of organic firm tofu (smoked tofu works well) instead of the chicken, stir-frying it in the same way.

CHICKEN SKEWERS WITH SATAY SAUCE

This is great in the summertime, perfect for cooking on the barbecue and a real crowd-pleaser if you're having a gathering! Pick a salad from pages 206–11 to serve with it, if you fancy. I like the Flu Slayer Salad – the toasted pumpkin seeds go especially well with this dish.

SERVES 1

1 LARGE CHICKEN BREAST, CUT INTO BITE-SIZE CHUNKS

150G CASHEWS

250G GOAT'S MILK YOGHURT

1 TSP DIJON MUSTARD

½ AN AVOCADO

1 Preheat the oven to 200°C/180°C fan/gas 6.

2 Slide the chicken pieces on to three wooden skewers. Place them on a baking tray and put into the oven for about 20 minutes.

3 Put the cashews, yoghurt and mustard into a food processor and blitz to a thick cream-like consistency.

4 When the chicken is crisp and cooked through, take it out of the oven and put it on a plate. Cut the avocado into bite-size pieces and add to the plate as well. Then pour the sauce over the chicken.

5 Go to the Salad section and pick one of the yummy salads! Serve it in a bowl alongside.

POST-TRAINING OPTION: Add a medium sweet potato, grilled, baked or made into fries (see page 227).

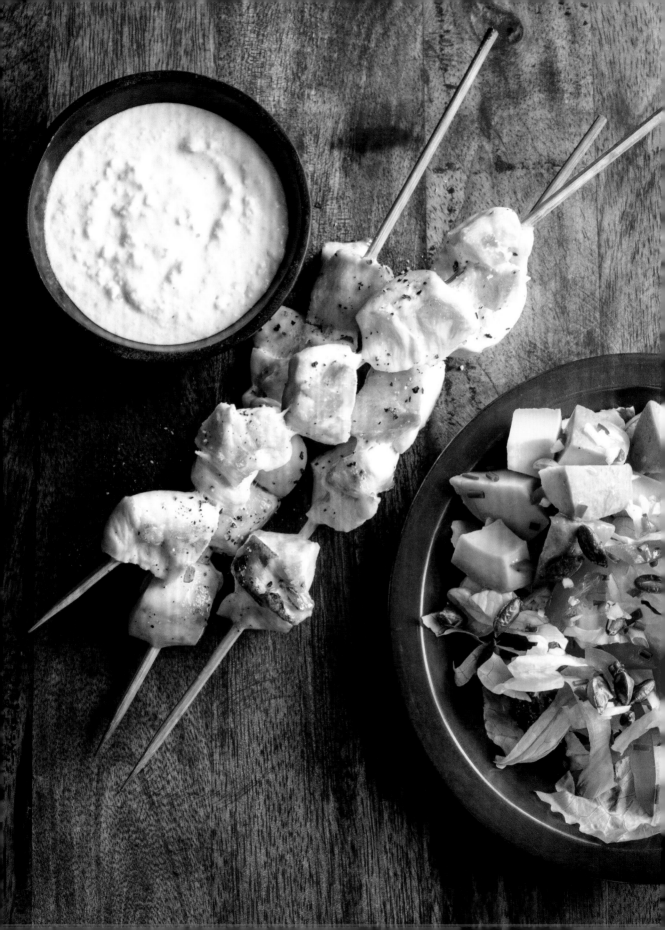

CHICKEN FLOWER SALAD

This salad is light but filling – a good one for when it's hot outside. I like to arrange it so it looks like a flower, with the lettuce, carrot and cucumber as the petals.

SERVES 1

1 TSP COCONUT OIL

1 LARGE CHICKEN BREAST,
CUT INTO BITE-SIZE PIECES

2 TSP PAPRIKA

SEA SALT AND FRESHLY
GROUND BLACK PEPPER

1 LITTLE GEM LETTUCE,
WASHED AND DRIED,
LARGE LEAVES HALVED

1 SMALL CARROT,
CUT INTO BATONS

½ A SMALL CUCUMBER,
CUT INTO BATONS

70G RED CABBAGE,
OUTER LEAVES REMOVED,
RINSED AND GRATED

1 TBSP HUMMUS

1 Put the oil into a pan and place on a medium heat. When hot, add the chicken, sprinkle over the paprika and season with salt and pepper. Cook, turning occasionally, for around 8 minutes, or until the chicken is fully cooked. Take off the heat and set aside.

2 Put the lettuce on a plate and arrange the carrot, cucumber and cabbage on top. Put the chicken in the middle and dot over the hummus.

POST-TRAINING: Sprinkle over a portion of Crunchy Roasted Chickpeas (see page 217).

COD WITH MEDITERRANEAN SPINACH & HALLOUMI

The texture and the flavour of the halloumi go perfectly with the cod and with the amazing immune-boosting side ingredients, garlic, spinach and lemon. Fish and cheese are not often paired, but I love fish and I love cheese. Vikings don't play by the rules.

SERVES 1

1 TSP COCONUT OIL

1–2 COD FILLETS
(I NORMALLY HAVE 2)

1 CLOVE OF GARLIC,
FINELY CHOPPED

4 SPRIGS OF FRESH THYME

JUICE OF 1 LEMON

SEA SALT AND FRESHLY
GROUND BLACK PEPPER

4 SLICES OF HALLOUMI
(ABOUT ½CM THICK)

2 TSP PAPRIKA

½ AN ONION, FINELY CHOPPED

6 CHERRY TOMATOES, HALVED

8 BLACK OLIVES, SLICED

70G SPINACH, WASHED

1 Preheat the oven to 220°C/200°C fan/gas 7.

2 Line a roasting tray with foil and spread over ½ teaspoon of the oil. Place the cod in the middle, sprinkle over the garlic and thyme, squeeze over the lemon juice and season with salt and pepper. Place the halloumi around the cod. Cook for 7 minutes, then take out and turn the halloumi over. Sprinkle over the paprika and return to the oven for another 6–8 minutes, or until the fish has turned opaque and can be easily flaked with a fork.

3 While the cod and halloumi are in the oven, put the remaining ½ teaspoon of coconut oil into a pan and place on a medium heat. Add the onion and fry for a couple of minutes, stirring. Add the tomatoes and olives and cook for a further few minutes, or until the tomatoes start to get soft and caramelize around the edges. Add a tiny splash of water to the pan and throw in the spinach. Stir until it wilts, then turn off the heat and serve alongside the cod and halloumi.

POST-TRAINING: Nutty barley goes really well with this dish. Soak 100g of barley overnight in water. Rinse, then put into a pan with 500ml of water. Bring to the boil, then reduce the heat and simmer for 45 minutes, or until cooked.

VEGGIE OPTION: Use 150g of organic tofu in place of the cod. Cut into strips lengthways and cook using the same method as for the cod. Cook for 15 minutes, then take out, flip over and add the halloumi and the paprika. Return to the oven for another 15 minutes.

HONEY GLAZED SALMON

Lemon pepper is my secret weapon for making all fish super yummy. (Well, that, plus butter.) In Iceland we use it quite a lot, though it seems less common in the UK. If you have lemon pepper and butter, then you are good. Add garlic salt and honey, and you are good as gold.

SERVES 1

1 TSP COCONUT OIL, OR
COLD-PRESSED RAPESEED OIL

1 SALMON FILLET
(APPROX. 140G)

LEMON PEPPER

GARLIC SALT

2 TSP RAW HONEY

40G SHEEP'S BUTTER,
CUT INTO SMALL PIECES

70G SPINACH, WASHED

½ AN AVOCADO

1 SMALL CARROT, PEELED

½ BEETROOT, PEELED

SEA SALT AND FRESHLY
GROUND BLACK PEPPER

A DRIZZLE OF OLIVE OIL

A SQUEEZE OF LEMON JUICE

1 Preheat the oven to 200°C/180°C fan/gas 6.

2 Line a roasting tray with a piece of foil large enough to wrap the fish, and spread the coconut oil over it. Place the salmon in the middle, and season with lemon pepper and garlic salt. Drizzle over the honey and dot with the butter, then fold the foil over and seal into a parcel. Roast for 15–20 minutes, adding the spinach to the tray for the last 5 minutes.

3 Cut the avocado into chunks and place in a medium-size bowl. Place a box grater over the top and coarsely grate in the carrot and beetroot (do the beetroot last, as its juice goes everywhere!). Season with salt and pepper, then mix it all together with a drizzle of olive oil and a squeeze of lemon.

4 Remove the salmon and spinach from the oven when ready, and serve with the salad alongside.

POST-TRAINING: Add 100g of cooked chickpeas to the crunchy side salad.

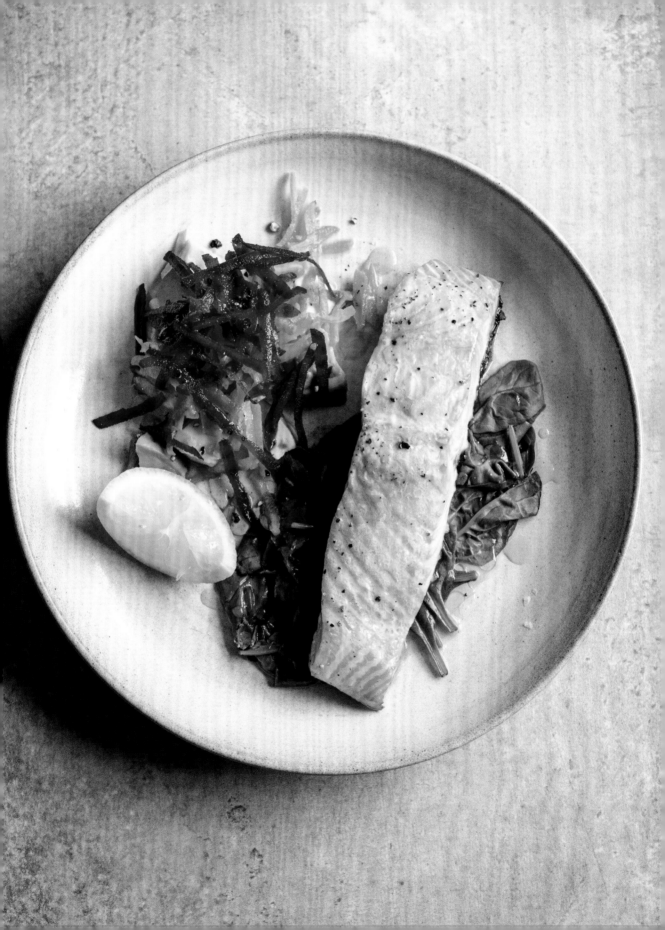

SESAME ARCTIC CHAR

This tastes fantastic and is so simple. Just the thing for evenings when you come home ravenous. Healthy fast food!

SERVES 1

1 TSP COCONUT OIL

2 ARCTIC CHAR FILLETS
(APPROX. 240G)

SEA SALT AND FRESHLY
GROUND BLACK PEPPER

1 TSP GARLIC SALT

100G SHEEP'S BUTTER

40ML SESAME OIL

40ML SWEET CHILLI SAUCE

1 TEASPOON SESAME SEEDS

5 SPRING ONIONS,
FINELY CHOPPED

1 CANTALOUPE MELON

1 Preheat the oven to 200°C/180°C fan/gas 6.

2 Take a roasting tray and spread the coconut oil over it. Place the Arctic char in the middle, and season with salt, pepper and the garlic salt.

3 Put the butter into a pan over a medium-low heat. Watch it carefully: remove from the heat when it is about three-quarters melted, and stir with a wooden spoon until completely melted. Mix in the sesame oil, chilli sauce, sesame seeds and spring onions, then pour over the char. Roast in the oven for 20 minutes. The fish should be easy to flake when it's done.

4 Peel the melon and take out the seeds. Cut into bite-size pieces and serve with the Arctic char.

POST-TRAINING: Add 100g of tinned butter beans. Drain and rinse the beans and put them into a pan for a few minutes over a low heat until they are warmed through. Drain and mix them in a bowl with the melon.

LAMB STEW

This is a proper Viking recipe, perfect for warming you up from the inside out on those long, cold winter nights. You can use any part of the lamb, but I like to use the leg. As a side, I really like to eat this with chopped tinned pears drizzled with a couple of teaspoons of melted raspberry jam. It might sound strange, but I love the sweetness with the rich, meaty lamb! The Alkaliner salad (see page 207) also goes really well.

SERVES 2–3

500G LAMB, CUT INTO BITE-SIZE PIECES

SEA SALT AND FRESHLY GROUND BLACK PEPPER

1 TBSP COLD-PRESSED RAPESEED OIL

2 ONIONS, FINELY CHOPPED

1 CLOVE OF GARLIC, FINELY CHOPPED

1 TBSP TOMATO PURÉE

½ TBSP PAPRIKA

2 BEEF STOCK CUBES, MIXED WITH 1 LITRE BOILING WATER

1 Season the lamb with salt and pepper.

2 Put the oil into a pan and place on a medium-high heat. When hot, add the lamb, browning it on all sides to seal it – around 5 minutes.

3 Transfer the lamb to a large heavy-bottomed pan, along with all the other ingredients. Bring to the boil, then reduce the heat, cover, and simmer for an hour, or until the meat is tender and in a rich savoury sauce.

POST-TRAINING: Serve with brown rice, to soak up all those good meaty juices.

VENISON SAUSAGES & SPICED BRAISED RED CABBAGE

Venison sausages are lean but full of flavour (just check the label and make sure they're not combined with pork), and are perfect with the sweet spiced cabbage.

SERVES 2

4 VENISON SAUSAGES

FOR THE RED CABBAGE

1 SMALL RED CABBAGE, CORE REMOVED, FINELY SLICED

1 RED GALA APPLE, CORED AND FINELY SLICED

½ A RED ONION, FINELY SLICED

1 TSP RAW HONEY

75ML CIDER VINEGAR

50ML RED WINE (OR WATER)

½ TSP JUNIPER BERRIES, LIGHTLY CRUSHED IN A PESTLE AND MORTAR

½ TSP GROUND CINNAMON

A KNOB OF GOAT'S BUTTER

SEA SALT AND FRESHLY GROUND BLACK PEPPER

1 Put all the red cabbage ingredients into a pan and place on a medium heat. Bring to a simmer, then turn the heat down slightly and cover with a lid. Cook for around 90 minutes, stirring occasionally, until the cabbage is fragrant and totally tender.

2 Preheat the oven to 200°C/180°C/gas 6. Line a roasting tray with foil and place a grill rack on top.

3 20 minutes before the cabbage is ready, put the sausages on to the grill rack and put the roasting tray into the oven. Roast until the sausages are dark golden and crisp, turning once or twice.

4 Serve the cabbage with the sausages.

VEGGIE OPTION: The braised cabbage is wonderful with goat's cheese melted on top. Just spoon the cabbage into an ovenproof dish, top with slices of goat's cheese, and bake at 180°C/160°C fan/gas 4 until melted and golden.

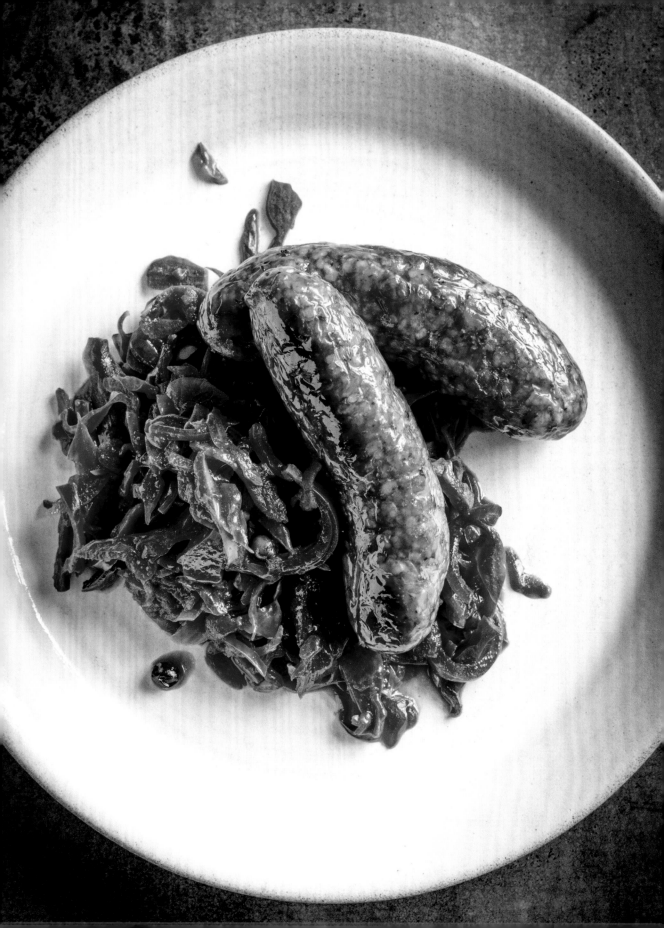

WHOLE ROASTED CELERIAC

This is an amazing vegetarian option – it couldn't be simpler to make, and any leftovers are great for your lunch box too. I like to serve this alongside a salad, or with kale or spinach, sautéd with garlic.

SERVES 4

1 WHOLE CELERIAC

1½ TBSP COLD-PRESSED RAPESEED OIL

2 TSP DIJON MUSTARD

1 TSP WHOLEGRAIN MUSTARD

4 CLOVES OF GARLIC, FINELY CHOPPED

4 SPRIGS OF FRESH THYME

A KNOB OF GOAT'S BUTTER, CHOPPED INTO SMALL PIECES

SEA SALT AND FRESHLY GROUND BLACK PEPPER

1 Preheat the oven to 200°C/180°C fan/gas 6. Line a baking tray with enough foil to entirely wrap the celeriac.

2 Scrub the celeriac well to remove any dirt or gnarly bits – a vegetable brush is handy if you have one. Make small incisions all over it with a sharp knife.

3 In a small bowl, mix together the oil, both mustards, garlic and thyme leaves (pull them off the sprigs) to make a marinade.

4 Place the celeriac in the middle of the tray and rub the marinade into it, really working to get it into the little cuts. Stud with the butter and season well with salt and pepper, then fold the foil over tightly to seal.

1 Roast for around 2 hours, or until completely tender, then slice into thick wedges and serve.

POST-TRAINING: Serve with a portion of cooked barley (see page 228).

LAMB GOULASH WITH BUTTERY MUSHROOMS

This is my mum's traditional Icelandic goulash. Just the thing to warm you up when it's cold outside and you've been giving it your all. Serve with a salad of your choice (see pages 206–11), or with my favourite – sautéd broccoli, red onion and tomatoes.

SERVES 2–3

500G LAMB (LEG OR SHOULDER WORK WELL, BUT YOU CAN USE ANY CUT)

A GOOD DRIZZLE OF COLD-PRESSED RAPESEED OIL

200ML WATER

1 BEEF STOCK CUBE

½ AN ONION, CHOPPED

100G ORGANIC TOMATO PURÉE

1–2 TBSP VEGAN, GOAT'S OR SHEEP'S BUTTER

200G WHITE BUTTON MUSHROOMS, CHOPPED

50G FRESH PARSLEY, CHOPPED

1 Preheat the oven to 180°C/160°C fan/gas 4.

2 Cut the lamb into chunks and place in a high-sided roasting tray. Drizzle with oil, turning the meat so that the pieces are all glazed. Roast for 20 minutes.

3 Put the water, beef stock cube, onion and tomato purée into a pan on a medium heat for a few minutes, mixing together to dissolve the stock cube.

4 Take the lamb out of the oven, pour over the beef stock mix and put back into the oven for 10 minutes.

5 Meanwhile put a pan on a medium heat and add the butter. Let it melt, then add the mushrooms. Stir them around in the butter until cooked and golden.

5 When the lamb is done, take it out of the oven and add the mushrooms, making sure to scrape in all the buttery juices. Sprinkle the chopped parsley over, and serve it up! (It is better to add the parsley at the end, as it is fully fresh and retains all its flavour.)

CREAMY CURRIED PEPPER SOUP

For those cosy nights in when you just want to relax and have it hygge, this hearty, healthy soup is perfect. Serve with a salad of your choosing (see pages 206–11).

SERVES 4

1 TSP COCONUT OIL

1 LEEK, WASHED WELL AND TRIMMED

4 PEPPERS (YELLOW, RED OR BOTH), DESEEDED AND CHOPPED

2 CLOVES OF GARLIC

1 TBSP ORGANIC CURRY PASTE

400G VEGAN CREAM CHEESE

180G CHILLI SAUCE

1 VEGETABLE STOCK CUBE, MIXED WITH 1½ LITRES BOILING WATER

250G DAIRY-FREE CREAM, SUCH AS SOYA OR COCONUT

GROUND PAPRIKA

SEA SALT AND FRESHLY GROUND BLACK PEPPER

1 Put the coconut oil into a pan (large enough for all the ingredients) and place on a medium heat. When hot, add the leeks to the pan and cook for a couple of minutes, stirring, until softened. Add the peppers, stir so everything is coated in oil, and cook for a couple more minutes.

2 Add the garlic and curry paste, stir well, and cook for 1 minute. Stir in the cream cheese, chilli sauce, stock, cream and paprika, and season with salt and pepper. Simmer gently for 5 minutes, stirring, to bring everything together.

3 Blend until smooth, using a hand-held electric blender.

OPTION: Chicken is really yummy in this soup. Cut chicken breasts (allow 1 per serving) into cubes and fry for 8–10 minutes in a little oil in a frying pan. Add to the soup at step 2, along with the other ingredients.

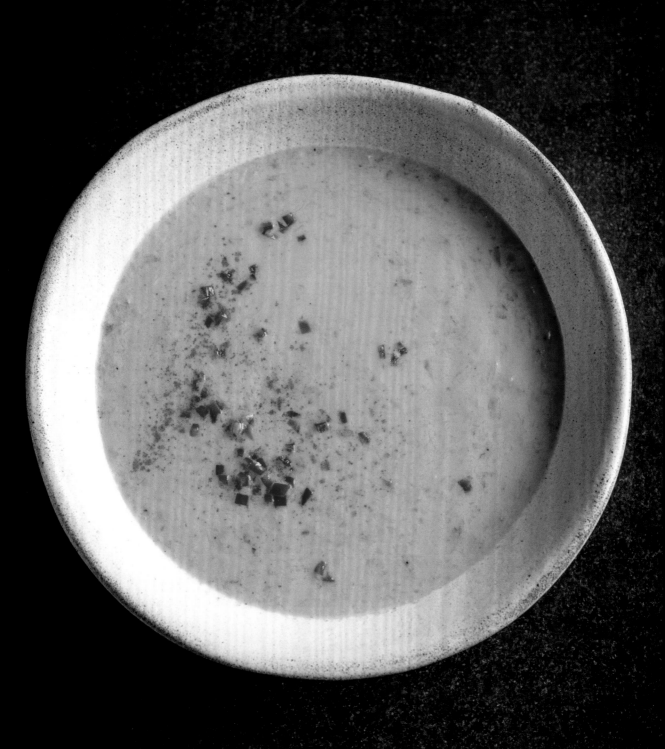

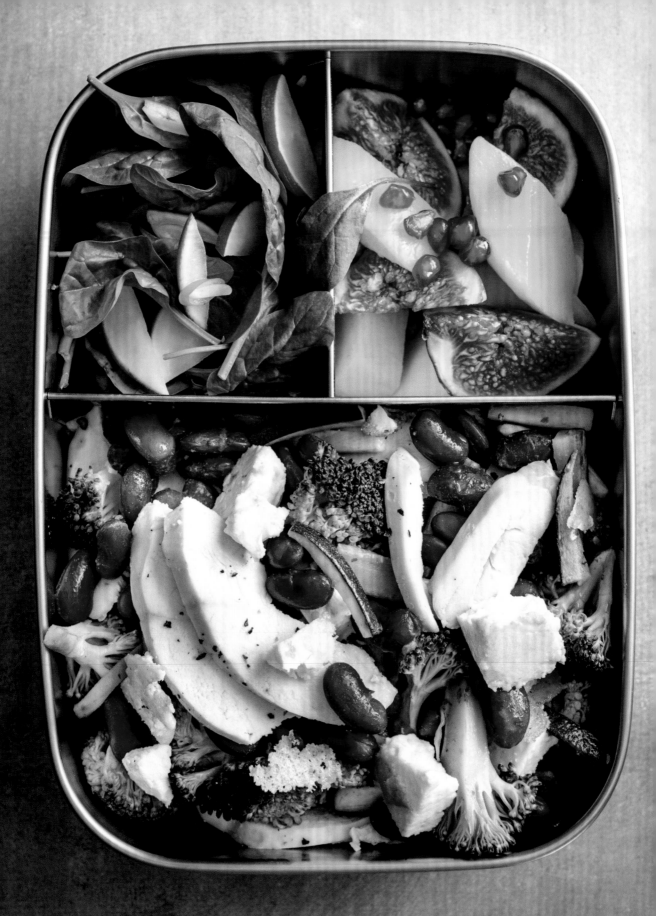

MY UGLY
LUNCH BOX

Lunch can be the most difficult meal of the day in terms of making healthy choices, especially if you're out and about with little time to eat or cook, and the easiest option is grabbing something quick and unhealthy.

If you turn to social media for inspiration you'll see pictures of perfectly packed lunches, all with perfectly aligned rainbow-coloured components, and rows of 'miracle' ingredients that are often only available in certain health food shops at a high price. Making a lunch like this can seem time-consuming and hard work, overly aspirational and ultimately off-putting. If you're anything like me, even if you bother to arrange everything perfectly in the morning, by the time you open your lunch box everything will be jumbled up together.

But that's OK. The Viking Method is about embracing our imperfections – and that extends to messy lunch boxes. Packed with the healthy nutrition you need to support you in your day, with ingredients you can get anywhere, the following lunches are tasty, quick and easy to make. Don't worry about killing yourself over the presentation: Ugly Lunch Boxes are all about the delicious contents!

Of course, you can make your lunch box the night before while you are cooking your dinner, but these recipes are so quick and simple you should be able to throw them together in the morning. Everyone's routine is different. I find it works best for me to either make an extra portion of dinner (like the Pesto Chicken & Sweet Potato One-tray Wonder, see page 124) or make my ugly box before I go to bed. If I leave it until the morning, I might not do it, as I always leave for work very early and don't want anything extra to do at the crack of dawn. Always know yourself and what works best for you.

There's also no reason why you shouldn't make these recipes for dinner instead – or why not make two portions, one for dinner and one for lunch the next day?

Remember to let the ingredients cool down before you put the lid on if you are doing your lunch box in the morning. If you place the lid on straight away it takes a lot longer to cool and you could be risking bacterial growth. Also, if you did prepare your box the night before, don't leave it behind in the fridge in your rush to get out of the door (we've all been there!).

POST-TRAINING LUNCH BOXES

Post-training lunch boxes are the same as other Post-training Meals – meant to be eaten on training days only, after you have worked out.

POST-TRAINING LUNCH BOXES
CHICKEN & FETA KIDNEY BEANS

A perfect example of what the Ugly Lunch Box is all about: quality on the inside! The feta and kidney beans taste amazing together, and your brain and nervous system will thank you for the vitamin K in the latter. Smarter with every bite!

SERVES 1

1 CHICKEN BREAST (COOKED, OR SEE METHOD FOR COOKING INSTRUCTIONS)

2 TSP COCONUT OIL

SEA SALT AND FRESHLY GROUND BLACK PEPPER

200G TINNED KIDNEY BEANS, DRAINED

½ A COURGETTE, SLICED INTO THIN MATCHSTICKS

6 BROCCOLI FLORETS

50G GOAT'S CHEESE FETA, CHOPPED INTO 1CM CUBES

1 If cooking the chicken from scratch, preheat the oven to 200°C/180°C fan/gas 6. Put the chicken in a foil-covered roasting tray, coat lightly with 1 teaspoon of coconut oil, and season with salt and pepper. Bake for 35 minutes, or until completely cooked through (slice into the thickest part to check, if you are unsure – the meat should be white and the juices clear). Remove and leave to cool, then slice into thin strips.

2 Put 1 teaspoon of coconut oil into a pan over a medium heat. When hot, add the kidney beans and courgettes and cook, stirring, for a few minutes, or until the courgettes soften and the beans begin to colour.

3 Add the broccoli to the pan for the last 2 minutes along with the feta – cook until the broccoli is just tender and the feta slightly melted.

4 Spoon into your lunch box and top with the chicken.

INDIAN-SPICED SALAD

This lunch box is probably the ugliest to date, but the warming combination of spices and beans is absolutely delicious, so what it lacks in looks it more than makes up for in flavour.

SERVES 1

100G DRIED BLACK TURTLE BEANS, SOAKED OVERNIGHT (SEE METHOD), OR USE TINNED BLACK BEANS

3 MEDIUM EGGS

1 TBSP COCONUT OIL

A LARGE THUMB-SIZE PIECE OF GINGER, PEELED AND GRATED

1 LARGE TOMATO, QUARTERED

½ TSP GROUND TURMERIC

½ TSP CORIANDER SEEDS

½ TSP CUMIN SEEDS

A HANDFUL OF SPINACH (150G), WASHED

SEA SALT AND FRESHLY GROUND BLACK PEPPER

1 If using dried beans, soak them overnight. Drain, put into a pan, then cover with fresh water and bring to the boil. Lower the heat to a simmer and cook for around 40 minutes, or until tender. Then drain them again. If using tinned beans, add them in step 4.

2 Fill a pan with enough cold water to cover the eggs and place on a medium to high heat. Once boiling, reduce the heat slightly and simmer for 3 minutes, then remove the eggs and place them in a bowl of cold water. Once cool, peel and halve the eggs (you could also do this just before eating, to minimize the 'eggy' smell of your lunch box, if you like).

3 Put the coconut oil into a pan and place on a high heat, then add the ginger and tomato. Mix together, then add the turmeric, and coriander and cumin seeds, and stir again.

4 Cook for a couple of minutes, then add the beans and spinach. If using tinned black beans, rinse and drain them before adding. Cook, stirring, until the spinach wilts, then remove from the heat and leave to cool down. Season with salt and pepper.

5 Spoon into your lunch box and top with the eggs.

TIP: I find that crushing the grated ginger with the back of a spoon helps to extract extra flavour from it – give it a go! Peel and grate the ginger, then use the back of a spoon to crush it completely, giving it a mashed consistency.

CHICKEN & BUTTERNUT SQUASH

This is one of my favourite lunch boxes. I find roast butternut squash absolutely delicious with chicken, and it has avocado. Sold!

SERVES 1

1 CHICKEN BREAST (COOKED, OR SEE METHOD FOR COOKING INSTRUCTIONS)

2 TSP COCONUT OIL

SEA SALT AND FRESHLY GROUND BLACK PEPPER

3 RINGS OF BUTTERNUT SQUASH, CUT INTO 1CM CUBES (CUT RINGS FROM THE THINNER END OF THE SQUASH)

1 LARGE CARROT, HALVED AND CUT INTO MATCHSTICKS

4 BROCCOLI FLORETS

1 SMALL AVOCADO

10 WHOLE RAW CASHEW NUTS, ROUGHLY CHOPPED, THEN CRUSHED

1 Preheat the oven to 200°C/180°C fan/gas 6.

2 If cooking the chicken from scratch, put it in a foil-covered roasting tray, coat lightly with 1 teaspoon of coconut oil and season with salt and pepper. Bake for 35 minutes, or until completely cooked through (slice into the thickest part to check, if you are unsure – the meat should be white and the juices clear). Remove and leave to cool, then slice into thin strips.

3 Line a second roasting tray with foil, add 1 teaspoon of coconut oil, then add the squash and carrots. Season with salt and pepper, then put into the oven and roast until soft, about 20 minutes. (Do this at the same time as the chicken, if cooking.) Add the broccoli for the last couple of minutes. Let the veg cool, then transfer to your lunch box.

4 Cut the avocado in half, carefully remove the stone (don't throw it out! You can use it for the Salmon with Avocado Stone, page 202), then, with the skin still on, cut a criss-cross pattern into each half and scoop out the flesh with a tablespoon.

5 To finish assembling your lunch box, add the chicken and avocado, and top with the cashews. Season with salt and pepper.

CHICKEN & LENTILS

The combination of lentils with the chicken stock, onion and thyme makes this juicy and rich in flavour.

SERVES 1

1 CHICKEN BREAST (COOKED, OR SEE METHOD FOR COOKING INSTRUCTIONS)

1 TSP COCONUT OIL

SEA SALT AND FRESHLY GROUND BLACK PEPPER

100G DRIED GREEN LENTILS

½ A CHICKEN STOCK CUBE

½ A SMALL ONION, FINELY CHOPPED

½ TSP DRIED THYME

1 SMALL CARROT, PEELED AND CHOPPED

70G KALE, WASHED

5 BROCCOLI FLORETS

1 SMALL AVOCADO

1 If cooking the chicken from scratch, preheat the oven to 200°C/180°C/gas 6. Put the chicken in a foil-covered roasting tray, coat lightly with coconut oil and season with salt and pepper. Bake for 35 minutes, or until completely cooked through (slice into the thickest part to check, if you are unsure – the meat should be white and the juices clear). Remove and leave to cool, then slice into thin strips.

2 Rinse the lentils, then put them into a small pan with 400ml of water. Place on a medium heat and bring to the boil, then lower the heat slightly and cook for 10 minutes. Add the chicken stock cube, onion and thyme and cook for another 10–15 minutes, until the lentils are tender but still have a tiny bite. Once done, leave them to cool.

3 Pour enough water to cover all the veg into another pan and bring to the boil. Once bubbling, add the carrots and cook for 3 minutes.

4 Add the kale and broccoli to the pan and cook for about 2 more minutes. Drain, then leave the veg to cool.

5 Cut the avocado in half, carefully remove the stone (don't throw it out! You can use it for the Salmon with Avocado Stone, page 202), then, with the skin still on, cut a criss-cross pattern into each half and scoop out the flesh with a tablespoon.

5 Assemble everything in your lunch box: lentils, veg, chicken, avocado. Boom!

ANYTIME LUNCH BOXES

You can change any of the Anytime lunch boxes into a Post-training lunch box by adding one of the Sometimes Carbs (see page 224–9).

ANYTIME LUNCH BOXES
TUNA, GREEN BEAN, ARTICHOKE & EGG SALAD

This is the simplest lunch ever, full of store-cupboard ingredients – so there is no excuse not to make it, even if you are feeling lazy or haven't had time to go shopping.

SERVES 1

3 MEDIUM EGGS

80G GREEN BEANS, TRIMMED AND HALVED

1 HEAD OF LITTLE GEM OR OTHER CRUNCHY LETTUCE, WASHED AND DRIED

80G TINNED ARTICHOKE HEARTS, CHOPPED

1 X 120G TIN OF TUNA IN SPRING WATER, DRAINED

50G GOAT'S MILK FETA, CHOPPED INTO 1CM CUBES

1 TBSP SUN-DRIED TOMATOES, FINELY CHOPPED

A DRIZZLE OF EXTRA VIRGIN OLIVE OIL

A DRIZZLE OF RED WINE VINEGAR

SEA SALT AND FRESHLY GROUND BLACK PEPPER

1 Put the eggs into a medium pan with enough cold water to cover them, and place on a medium to high heat. Once boiling, add the green beans, reduce the heat slightly and simmer for 3 minutes. Remove the eggs and beans and place them in a bowl of cold water. Once cool, peel and halve the eggs (you could also do this just before eating, to minimize the 'eggy' smell of your lunch box, if you like) and drain the beans.

2 Chop the lettuce if the leaves are big and place in your lunch box followed by the green beans, artichokes, tuna, feta and sun-dried tomatoes. Drizzle with oil and vinegar, season with salt and pepper, and top with the eggs.

SALMON & SUPER GREENS

It doesn't get much better than this heavenly green box, packed with antioxidants, healthy fats, vitamins and minerals. It ticks all the boxes when it comes to getting as much goodness into you as possible in one meal, and flavourwise, the oily, buttery salmon is perfectly offset by the earthy beetroot.

SERVES 1

1 SMALL UNCOOKED BEETROOT

1 SALMON FILLET

A KNOB OF GOAT'S BUTTER, SOFT ENOUGH TO SPREAD

1 TBSP COCONUT OIL, OR COLD-PRESSED RAPESEED OIL

4 SPRING ONIONS, CHOPPED

1 CLOVE OF GARLIC, CRUSHED

A HANDFUL OF KALE, WOODY STALKS REMOVED, ROUGHLY CHOPPED

4 BROCCOLI FLORETS

½ AN AVOCADO, CHOPPED

SEA SALT AND FRESHLY GROUND BLACK PEPPER

A SQUEEZE OF LEMON JUICE (OPTIONAL)

1 Wash and trim the beetroot, then place it in a saucepan and cover with water. Put on a high heat and bring to the boil, then lower the heat to medium and cook for 30 minutes until cooked through (poke with a small knife or toothpick to check). Leave to cool, then push the skin off with your hands and slice into ¼cm rounds.

2 Preheat the oven to 200°C/180°C fan/gas 6. Line a baking tray with a piece of foil large enough to wrap the salmon. Place the salmon in the tray and cover with the goat's butter. Close the foil on top. Bake for 15 minutes.

3 Heat the oil in a frying pan on a medium heat, then add the spring onions and garlic and cook for a couple of minutes, until softened.

4 Add the sliced beetroot, kale and broccoli and cook for another 2 minutes, or until just tender.

5 Remove the salmon from the oven, leave to cool, then put into the ugly box along with the avocado and the veggies. Season with salt and pepper, and squeeze over some lemon juice, if you like.

TIP: Prep ahead and give yourself a hand by cooking a bunch of beetroots at the same time. Cover or store in an airtight container and leave in the fridge until you need them. Here are few of the recipes that contain beetroot: Speedy Viking Smörgåsbord (page 119), Chicken with Curried Scrambled Eggs, Lentils & Good Stuff (page 127), Honey Glazed Salmon (page 182).

GREEN AVO EGGS

Fantastic healthy meals don't get simpler than this – so why complicate things?

SERVES 1

3 MEDIUM EGGS

5 BROCCOLI FLORETS

A HANDFUL OF SPINACH
(ROUGHLY 150G), WASHED

1 SMALL AVOCADO

40G GOAT'S MILK FETA,
CUT INTO CUBES

SEA SALT AND FRESHLY
GROUND BLACK PEPPER

1 Put the eggs into a pan with enough cold water to cover them, and place on a medium to high heat. Once boiling, reduce the heat slightly and simmer for 3 minutes, then remove the eggs and place them in a bowl of cold water. Once cool, peel and halve the eggs (you could also do this just before eating, to minimize the 'eggy' smell of your lunch box, if you like).

2 Place a couple of pieces of kitchen paper on a clean chopping board. While the eggs are on the go, fill another pan with water (salt it if you like), and bring to the boil. Once bubbling, add the broccoli and cook for a couple of minutes, or until just tender. Remove with a slotted spoon and leave on the kitchen paper to drain. Next, add the spinach, blanch for 30 seconds, then again remove with a slotted spoon and leave to drain.

3 Cut the avocado in half, carefully remove the stone, then, with the skin still on, cut a criss-cross pattern into each half and scoop out the flesh with a tablespoon.

4 Combine all the ingredients in your lunch box and season with salt and pepper.

TIP: Again, help yourself by boiling several eggs and keeping them in the fridge ready for whenever you need them (kept in their shells, freshly boiled eggs should be good for up to one week). I do this and it makes such a difference! It isn't just the boy scouts who are always prepared, it's also us Vikings!

SALMON WITH AVOCADO STONE

Yes, I really do mean an avocado stone, the middle of the avocado that usually ends up in the bin. Making use of it is the kind of thing I love, a little thing that makes such a big difference. So, why use the avocado stone? It's high in antioxidants and anti-inflammatories, properties purported to aid in maintaining healthy digestion, skin elasticity, circulation and good heart health. With all the recipes that use an avocado, take the stone out and place in the fridge. After it has dried, which takes about 3 days, it is ready to be grated over your meals.

SERVES 1

1 AVOCADO STONE, LEFT IN THE FRIDGE FOR 3 DAYS TO DRY OUT (SAVE ONE FROM EARLIER IN THE WEEK!)

1 SALMON FILLET

SEA SALT AND FRESHLY GROUND BLACK PEPPER

1 TSP DRIED OREGANO

1 TBSP COCONUT OIL

½ YELLOW OR RED PEPPER, DESEEDED AND SLICED

4 BROCCOLI FLORETS

3 CHERRY TOMATOES, HALVED

1 SMALL AVOCADO

50G GOAT'S MILK FETA, CUT INTO 1CM CHUNKS

1 LEMON

1 To prepare the avocado stone, cut off the outer layer, throw that away, then use a cheese grater to grate the remaining part of the stone. I use about a quarter of it, but you can use as much as you want.

2 Preheat the oven to 200°C/180°C fan/gas mark 6.

3 Line a baking tray with a piece of tin foil large enough to totally wrap the salmon. Place the salmon in the centre of the foil and season with salt, pepper and the oregano.

4 Put the coconut oil into a pan over a medium heat and, when hot, add the yellow or red pepper and cook for 2–3 minutes, stirring occasionally until softened.

5 Add the broccoli and cook for a further couple of minutes, until just tender, then add the tomatoes and cook for a minute more.

6 Halve the avocado and carefully remove the stone (don't throw it out – keep it for grating next time – see above). Then, with the skin still on, cut a criss-cross pattern into each half and scoop out the flesh with a tablespoon.

7 Assemble your lunch box: start with the veggies from the pan, then the salmon fillet, and finish with the avocado and feta. Lastly, cut the lemon in half and squeeze the juice over, then add the grated avocado stone and stir.

TIP: I tend to prep the most time-consuming part of my Ugly Lunch Box the night before (if I'm not using up any leftovers from a previous dinner) or in a batch – anything that needs time in the oven, like raw fish and chicken, or boiling, such as eggs and Sometimes Carbs (see pages 224–9). This way, it's manageable to do everything else quickly right before you go to bed or first thing in the morning.

CHICKEN WITH MUSHROOMS & GINGER

Fresh ginger is such a health chief. It's been suggested that it can improve brain function and help fight infection, in addition to its traditionally recognized restorative properties which can range from soothing digestion and inflammation, to reducing muscle pain, to alleviating nausea – particularly morning sickness. It tastes wonderfully pungent and spicy too, so pack it into your lunch!

SERVES 1

1 CHICKEN BREAST
(COOKED, OR SEE METHOD
FOR COOKING INSTRUCTIONS)

1 TBSP COCONUT OIL,
PLUS 1 TSP

SEA SALT AND FRESHLY
GROUND BLACK PEPPER

5 CLOSED-CUP MUSHROOMS,
SLICED

A THUMB-SIZE PIECE OF
GINGER, GRATED

1 CLOVE OF GARLIC, CRUSHED

A LARGE HANDFUL (150G)
OF SPINACH, WASHED

1 SMALL AVOCADO

JUICE OF ½ A LIME (OPTIONAL)

A DRIZZLE OF SESAME OIL
(OPTIONAL)

1 If cooking the chicken from scratch, preheat the oven to 200°C/180°C fan/gas 6. Put the chicken on a foil-covered roasting tray, coat lightly with 1 teaspoon of coconut oil and season with salt and pepper. Bake for 35 minutes, or until completely cooked through (slice into the thickest part to check, if you are unsure – the meat should be white and the juices clear). Remove and leave to cool. Then slice the chicken into thin strips.

2 Put a tablespoon of coconut oil into a pan over a medium heat, and when hot, add the mushrooms, ginger and garlic and cook, stirring occasionally, for about 2 minutes, until softened and slightly golden.

3 Add the spinach to the pan and cook until wilted.

4 Cut the avocado in half, carefully remove the stone, then, with the skin still on, slice each half lengthways and scoop out the flesh with a tablespoon.

5 Put all the ingredients into your lunch box: they'll get jumbled up, but I like to start with a layer of the ginger-garlic spinach and mushrooms, and finish with the sliced chicken and avocado slices. Season with salt and pepper to taste, and finish with a squeeze of lime juice and a drizzle of sesame oil if you like.

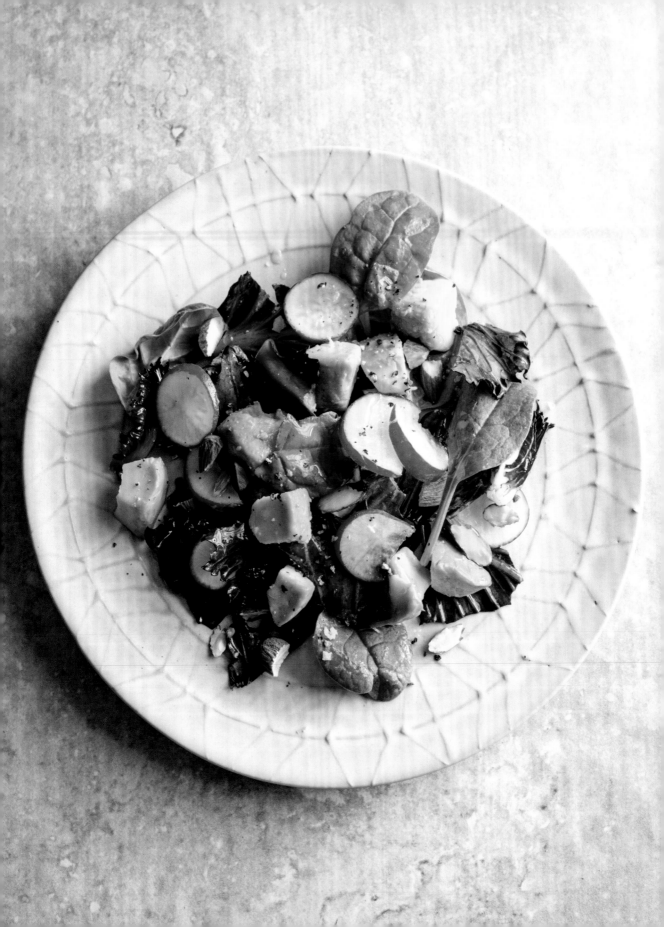

SALADS,
SAUCES
AND
SNACKS

SALADS (ANYTIME)

Whether it's a training day or not, these salads are a delicious way to top up your five-a-day.

Enjoy alongside any of the main meals as a side salad. Or add protein such as sliced chicken, turkey, egg, flaked fish, sliced tofu, or a handful of cooked lentils or beans, and make it into a main meal.

If it's a training day and you want a salad as a main meal, add a portion of Sometimes Carbs (see pages 224–9).

I have suggested my favourite combinations below, but how much you use of each ingredient is up to you. If you are having a salad as a main meal, you will likely want to use more – 150g of spinach rather than 80g, say. Everything in these salads is healthy and good for you, so you really can't go wrong (unless you use 15 chillies!).

Dress with extra virgin olive oil and a squeeze of lemon juice, either drizzled straight over the salad, or whisked together in a small bowl with salt and pepper. If you like mustard, you could add ¼ teaspoon of that too, or turn to the Sauces on pages 212–5 for inspiration.

THE INFLAMMATION WARRIOR

Anti-inflammatory foods are pure gold, boosting your immune system, and keeping you fighting fit! Carrots, red onions and beetroots are all great warriors against inflammation.

SERVES 1

CARROT, JULIENNED

RED CABBAGE, SHREDDED

BLACK OLIVES, CHOPPED

RED ONION, THINLY SLICED

COOKED BEETROOT, SLICED

MAIN OPTION: Add 120g of drained tinned tuna.

SOMETIMES CARB: Green or brown lentils.

THE ALKALINER

Too much acid causes absolute havoc in your body, negatively affecting your bones, skin, digestion and joints, among other things. Therefore it is important to get nutrients in that balance out the acid and keep it from getting too high. Dark leafy greens, radishes, avocado and almonds are all alkaline foods.

SERVES 1

AVOCADO, PEELED AND CUT INTO CHUNKS

BABY SPINACH, WASHED

RADISHES, SLICED

ALMONDS, ROUGHLY CHOPPED

KALE, WASHED AND RIPPED INTO PIECES

MAIN OPTION: Add a sliced chicken breast: preheat the oven to 200°C/180°C fan/gas 6. Put 1 large chicken breast on a foil-covered tray, coat lightly with rapeseed or coconut oil, and season with salt and pepper. Roast for 35 minutes, or until completely cooked, then take out of the oven and leave to cool slightly before slicing.

SOMETIMES CARB: Quinoa.

THE POTASSIUM SOLDIER

Potassium is an electrolyte that is crucial to good heart function as well as playing a key role in muscle contraction, making it important for good skeletal and muscular function. Spinach and cherry tomatoes are both great sources of potassium. If you have time, toast the pine nuts in a dry frying pan: it really adds to the flavour.

SERVES 1

BABY SPINACH, WASHED

RED ONION, THINLY SLICED

CHERRY TOMATOES, HALVED

PINE NUTS

FRESH BASIL

MAIN OPTION: Add 100g of sliced halloumi, fried with a drizzle of rapeseed oil in a non-stick pan until golden.

SOMETIMES CARB: Cooked barley.

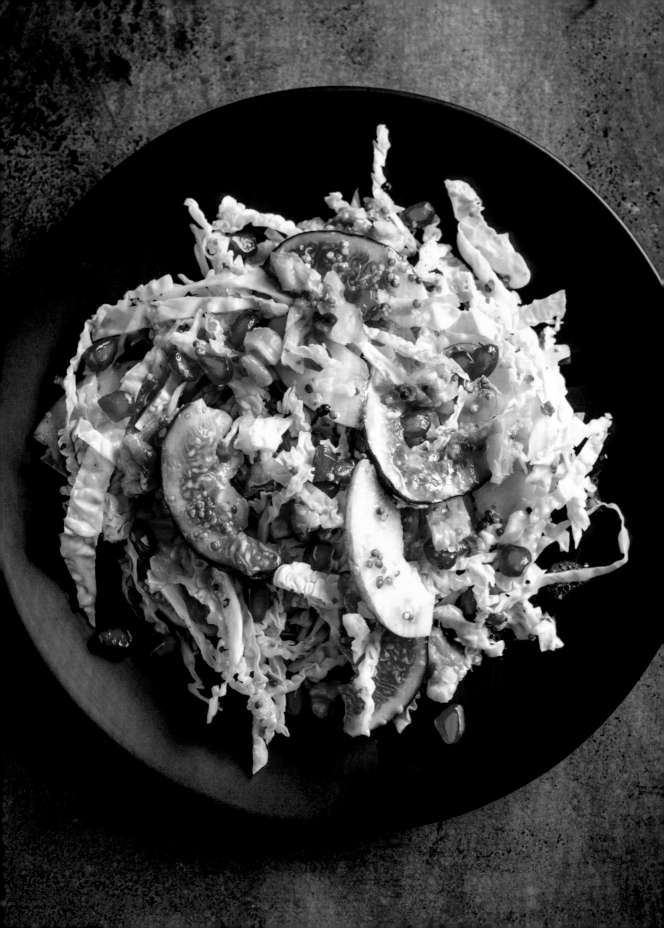

THE BONE STRENGTHENER

All the ingredients in this salad help to keep your bones strong: calcium, vitamin C, magnesium, and flavonoids that increase their density. Vikings need to have extremely strong bones, obviously, to be ready for berserkness!

SERVES 1

GREEN CABBAGE, SHREDDED

APPLE, CORED AND
THINLY SLICED

WALNUTS, CHOPPED

FIGS, TOPS TRIMMED,
CUT INTO WEDGES

POMEGRANATE SEEDS

MAIN OPTION: Add a flaked smoked mackerel fillet.

SOMETIMES CARB: Brown rice.

THE FLU SLAYER

Take good care of your immune system, feeding it with soldiers that kill any flu wishers: all the ingredients here do exactly that, keeping your immune system at optimum level with their natural immune-boosting, antioxidant, anti-inflammatory, de-stressing components. This salad calls for a super potent dressing: in a bowl mix together a drizzle of oil with the juice of a whole lemon and add a grated garlic clove and the chilli.

SERVES 1

ROMAINE LETTUCE,
WASHED AND CHOPPED

RED PEPPERS, DESEEDED
AND SLICED

CHIVES, FINELY CHOPPED

PUMPKIN SEEDS, TOASTED

LEMON JUICE

1 CLOVE OF GARLIC, FINELY
GRATED OR CRUSHED

RED CHILLI, DESEEDED
AND FINELY SLICED

MAIN OPTION: Add 150g of cooked king prawns.

SOMETIMES CARB: Vermicelli rice noodles.

THE ANTIOXIDANT

Antioxidants fight against cell damage caused by free radicals: melon, tomatoes, kale, red peppers and cucumber are all high in antioxidants. To tenderize raw kale, put it into a bowl with a drizzle of oil and lemon juice and a pinch of salt, and massage the dressing into the leaves with your hands. Leave for 10 minutes while you prepare the other ingredients.

SERVES 1

MELON, CUT INTO CHUNKS

KALE, WASHED AND RIPPED INTO PIECES

CHERRY TOMATOES, HALVED

RED PEPPER, DESEEDED AND FINELY SLICED

CUCUMBER, SLICED INTO HALF MOONS

MAIN OPTION: Add a seared tuna steak: preheat a pan on medium to high heat, brush the tuna steak with rapeseed oil and season on both sides with salt and pepper. Add to the pan and cook for 2–2½ minutes on each side.

SOMETIMES CARB: Egg noodles.

THE DE-STRESSER

The negative effects of stress and anxiety on your body and on your mental health are severe. Foods rich in B vitamins are an excellent way to bring calmness and help to de-stress. Gem lettuce, broccoli, goat's milk feta and red pepper are all fantastic sources of B vitamins, which calm the nervous system.

SERVES 1

LITTLE GEM LETTUCE, TRIMMED AND LEAVES WASHED

BROCCOLI, ROUGHLY CHOPPED

GOAT'S MILK FETA, CRUMBLED

CHERRY TOMATOES, HALVED

SUNFLOWER SEEDS (TOASTED, IF YOU LIKE)

RED PEPPER, DESEEDED AND FINELY SLICED

MAIN OPTION: Add sliced steak: brush the steak with a little rapeseed oil and season on both sides with salt and pepper, then cook in a hot pan for 3–4 minutes on each side for medium. Remove and leave to rest before slicing. For greater details on how to cook steak, go to the recipe for Sirloin Steak with Filled Portobello Mushrooms on page 178.

SOMETIMES CARB: A baked sweet potato.

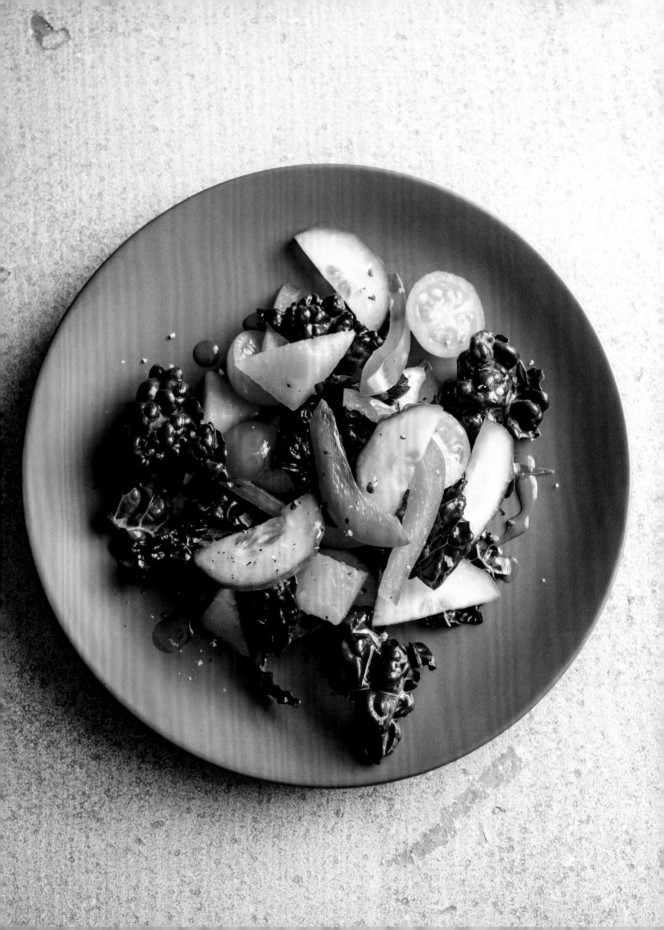

SAUCES

Healthy sauces can be tricky to buy ready-made (as they are often full of sugar), so I generally find it easier to make my own. Everyone has their own unique tastes and preferences – that's why all my recipes allow you to swap in your favourite flavours and ingredients with just a little bit of guidance.

You could add any of these sauces to wraps (pages 152–7), serve them alongside a main meal, or drizzle them over your lunch box. Whatever you do, you are nourishing your body with healthy ingredients.

Each of these recipes is enough for 3–4 people, but any leftovers can be stored in the fridge for 3 days.

RAITA CUCUMBER SAUCE

1 CUCUMBER, CHOPPED VERY FINELY

1 TSP CUMIN SEEDS, CRUSHED IN A PESTLE AND MORTAR (IF YOU DON'T HAVE A PESTLE AND MORTAR, PLACE THEM ON A STABLE CHOPPING BOARD, PLACE A HEAVY POT ON TOP OF THEM AND SLOWLY MOVE IT OVER THE SEEDS)

400ML GOAT'S MILK YOGHURT

2 TBSP FRESH CORIANDER

A SPRINKLE OF GROUND CAYENNE PEPPER

SEA SALT AND FRESHLY GROUND BLACK PEPPER

Put all the ingredients into a blender (or a large bowl if you are using a hand blender).

Blitz to combine, and season with salt and pepper to taste.

TURMERIC YOGHURT SAUCE

250ML GOAT'S MILK YOGHURT

1 TSP GRATED FRESH TURMERIC

½ A CLOVE OF GARLIC

1 TSP ORGANIC RAW HONEY

SEA SALT AND FRESHLY GROUND BLACK PEPPER

Put all the ingredients into a blender (or a large bowl if you are using a hand blender).

Blitz to combine, and season with salt and pepper to taste.

YOGHURT PESTO SAUCE

150ML GOAT'S MILK YOGHURT

150G PESTO (JARRED IS FINE, JUST CHECK THE INGREDIENTS: THERE SHOULD BE NO HARD COW'S CHEESE AND LESS THAN 5G SUGAR PER 100G)

1 TSP ORGANIC RAW HONEY

SEA SALT AND FRESHLY GROUND BLACK PEPPER

Put all the ingredients into a blender (or a large bowl if you are using a hand blender).

Blitz to combine, and season with sea salt and freshly ground black pepper to taste.

AVOCADO SAUCE

4 TBSP EXTRA VIRGIN OLIVE OIL

1 CLOVE OF GARLIC, CRUSHED

1 TSP PINE NUTS

1 AVOCADO, MASHED

SEA SALT AND FRESHLY GROUND BLACK PEPPER

Put all the ingredients into a blender (or a large bowl if you are using a hand blender).

Blitz to combine, then add a little water until it has a thick but sauce-like consistency. Season with salt and pepper to taste.

GINGER & HERB DRESSING

This dressing will keep in the fridge for up to a week.

1 CLOVE OF GARLIC, CHOPPED

A MEDIUM KNOB OF GINGER, GRATED

½ A SHALLOT, FINELY CHOPPED

½ A RED CHILLI, DESEEDED AND CHOPPED

JUICE OF 1 LEMON

25G MIX OF FRESH PARSLEY AND DILL

240ML EXTRA VIRGIN OLIVE OIL

SEA SALT AND FRESHLY GROUND BLACK PEPPER

Put all the ingredients into a blender (or a large bowl if you are using a hand blender).

Blitz to combine, and season with salt and pepper to taste.

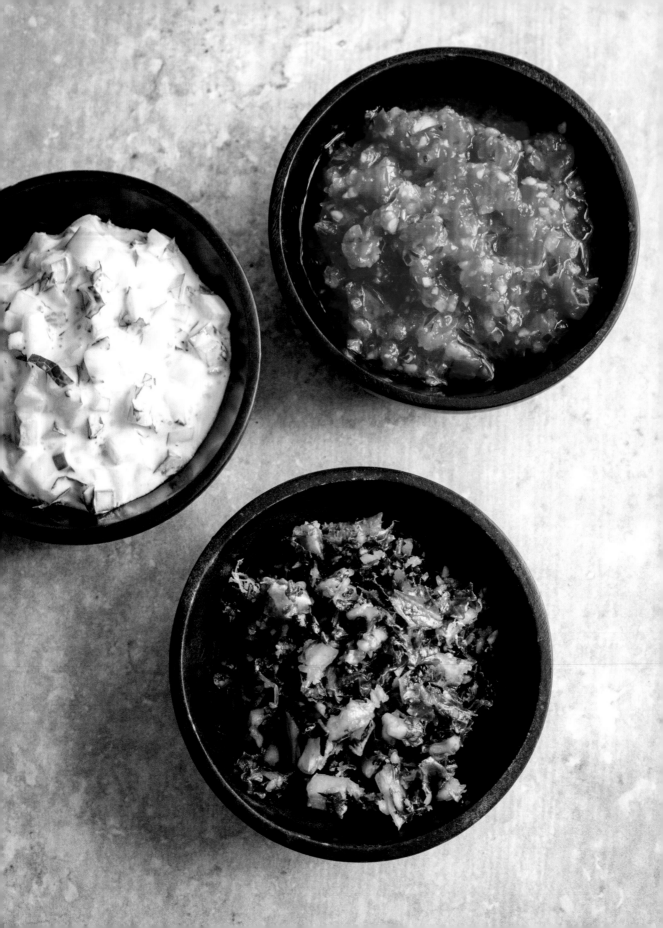

TZATZIKI

350ML GOAT'S MILK YOGHURT

1 CUCUMBER, CHOPPED VERY FINELY

2 CLOVES OF GARLIC, CRUSHED

1 TBSP EXTRA VIRGIN OLIVE OIL

A HANDFUL OF FRESH HERBS, SUCH AS MINT
OR DILL, ROUGHLY CHOPPED

SEA SALT AND FRESHLY GROUND BLACK PEPPER

Put all the ingredients into a bowl and
mix together. Season with salt and pepper
to taste.

FRESH SALSA

3 TOMATOES, CHOPPED

½ A RED ONION, CHOPPED

1 CLOVE OF GARLIC, CHOPPED

1 TBSP RICE WINE VINEGAR

½ TSP PAPRIKA

SEA SALT AND FRESHLY GROUND BLACK PEPPER

Put all the ingredients into a bowl and
mix together. Season with salt and pepper
to taste.

KALE & WALNUT PESTO

This rich, zingy pesto is packed full of nutrient-rich dark greens, with walnuts providing those essential omega-3s. Pecorino is of course made with sheep's milk. All the good stuff! Use this pesto in the Speltotto (see page 129). The recipe here will make one jar, which should keep, sealed, in the fridge for up to a week.

100G WALNUTS

250G CURLY KALE, ANY THICK WOODY STEMS
REMOVED, LEAVES ROUGHLY CHOPPED

50G PECORINO CHEESE, GRATED

2 CLOVES OF GARLIC

JUICE AND ZEST OF ½ A LEMON

3 TBSP COLD-PRESSED RAPESEED OIL

SEA SALT AND FRESHLY GROUND BLACK PEPPER

Put a pan on a low-medium heat and add the walnuts. Toast for a couple of minutes, stirring occasionally, until they colour ever so slightly and smell fragrant and nutty. Remove from the heat immediately and leave to cool.

Put the kale, pecorino, garlic, lemon zest, oil and walnuts into a food processor or small hand mixer and blend. Add the lemon juice a splash at a time until it reaches the right sauce-y but not too runny pesto consistency. Season with salt and pepper to taste.

SNACKS

There's a misconception that snacking is bad, but it's really important to make sure you have something nutritious to nibble on when hunger strikes. I always make sure I have something to hand so I'm not caught out. It doesn't need to be complicated or time-consuming – sometimes it might just be a few carrot sticks, or a boiled egg (the most perfectly portable snack, with its protective shell), or a handful of your favourite nuts.

If you're at home, or have access to a kitchen, a tasty quick snack might be an apple, sliced, with a little ground cinnamon sprinkled over it, or some lovely crunchy vegetables like carrot, celery or cucumber sticks, or radishes (allow 6 per portion) with hummus. You don't have to make your own hummus: there are many great organic varieties readily available. Always check the sugar content: it should be lower than 5g per 100g. If you want to jazz up store-bought hummus, add a drizzle of Kale & Walnut Pesto (see page 215), a sprinkling of toasted pumpkin seeds, or even just a pinch of smoky paprika.

Apart from the Crunchy Roasted Chickpeas, all snacks can be enjoyed on Rest or Training Days.

KALE AND SEAWEED CRISPS

It's thought that a traditional Viking diet would have included seaweed – not surprising when you think how much time was spent in those longboats! Full of nutrients and umami-rich, these seaweed crisps are a tasty snack and another way to eat your greens.

SERVES 4

40G DULSE (SEAWEED)

250G CURLY KALE, THICK WOODY STEMS REMOVED, LEAVES TORN INTO BITE-SIZE PIECES

2 TSP RAPESEED OIL

A GOOD PINCH OF SMOKED SEA SALT

A GOOD PINCH OF SMOKED PAPRIKA

1 Preheat the oven to 170°C/150°C fan/gas 3.

2 Place the dulse in a small bowl and cover with boiling water. Leave for a couple of minutes to soften and rehydrate, then drain, pat dry and chop into small pieces.

3 Line a baking tray with foil, add the kale and dulse, then drizzle over the oil and sprinkle over the sea salt and paprika. Toss, massaging the oil and seasoning into the leaves with your hands – you want to make sure everything is evenly coated, so work it!

4 Bake in the oven for 5 minutes, then shake the tray and return it to the oven for a couple more minutes, until the kale and dulse are crisp and slightly browned at the edges.

5 Remove and adjust the seasoning to taste if you feel it needs more. Any leftovers will keep in a sealed Tupperware box or other airtight container for a couple of days.

CRUNCHY ROASTED CHICKPEAS

The perfect training day snack for replenishing your carbs and energy. These are also great added to a main meal eaten post-training, particularly the Cajun-spiced Chicken with Halloumi (see page 163) and the Chicken & Golden Cauliflower Rice (see page 164).

SERVES 4

1 TSP COCONUT OIL, OR COLD-PRESSED RAPESEED OIL

1 X 400G TIN OF CHICKPEAS, WELL DRAINED

SEA SALT FLAKES

SPICES: GARAM MASALA AND GROUND TURMERIC/GARLIC SALT AND FENNEL SEEDS/ GROUND CINNAMON AND CUMIN SEEDS/SMOKY PAPRIKA AND CHILLI FLAKES (OR TRY YOUR OWN COMBINATIONS OF SPICES)

1 Preheat the oven to 200°C/180°C fan/gas 6.

2 Pat the drained chickpeas dry with kitchen paper, as they will take longer to crisp up if they are too wet. Drizzle the oil on a baking tray, add the chickpeas and mix well.

3 Season with flaky sea salt and season generously with your choice of spices.

4 Roast for 35 minutes, stirring the chickpeas a couple of times to turn them over, until they are evenly and properly crispy.

VIKING BALLER BALLS

These chewy, flavour-packed balls are filled with energy to ensure you keep up your strength, while avoiding the extra hidden sugary ingredients so many shop-bought balls and bars contain. We Vikings like them clean and powerful! Team with Odin's Green & Mean smoothie (see page 223) for the ultimate slayer snack!

MAKES ABOUT 8 BALLS (1 BALL = 1 SERVING)

200G ALMONDS

150G SHELLED HEMP SEEDS

70G CASHEWS

60G ALMOND MILK

2 TSP CACAO POWDER

30G COCONUT FLAKES

1 TSP GROUND CINNAMON

1 Put all the ingredients into a food processor and blitz until everything is well combined and has a soft paste-like consistency.

2 Scoop the mixture out of the processor and roll portions between your hands to make the balls. Each should be around the size of a large golfball, and you should end up with about 8 balls.

3 Place the balls in a Tupperware box or other airtight container and leave in the fridge to set for at least an hour.

LOLLIES

These are amazing as a snack and perfect when you get those sweet cravings in the evening. Ice lollies are so popular in Iceland, and my mum started making healthy lollies with me and my siblings when we were younger, so that we could get in all the good stuff that kids often say no to. We loved them in the summer as well as on cold Icelandic winter nights – we Vikings are hardy! All these lollies give you loads of strength, vitality and health goodness. Viking weapons against illnesses, low energy, internal stress and injuries.

Each recipe makes 4 lollies.

FREYR'S SWORD

Freyr is the god of health, abundance and prosperity, said to be 'the foremost of the gods and hated by none'.

1CM THICK SLICE OF PINEAPPLE, ROUGHLY CHOPPED

1 SMALL RED GALA APPLE, SKIN ON, ROUGHLY CHOPPED

70G MANGO, PEELED AND ROUGHLY CHOPPED

1 KIWI, PEELED AND ROUGHLY CHOPPED

FORSETI'S GOLDEN AXE

Forseti is the god of justice, mediation and reconciliation, and greatly respected. The word 'forseti' in Icelandic means president, and is used as such.

1 PLUM, STONED AND ROUGHLY CHOPPED

1 TBSP PUMPKIN AND SUNFLOWER SEEDS

1 APPLE, SKIN ON, ROUGHLY CHOPPED

½ A COOKED BEETROOT, ROUGHLY CHOPPED

6 STRAWBERRIES, TOPS CUT OFF AND HALVED

THOR'S HAMMER

½ AN AVOCADO

1 TSP FLAXSEEDS

1 TSP GOJI BERRIES

7 STRAWBERRIES, TOPS CUT OFF AND HALVED

70G BLUEBERRIES

ODIN'S SPEAR

1 AVOCADO, PEELED AND ROUGHLY CHOPPED

125G RASPBERRIES

A HANDFUL OF CASHEWS

Put all the ingredients into a food processor (chopping any that need to be chopped beforehand) and blitz together. Add a splash of water at the end if needed, but only a little. The consistency should be thick, like soft ice cream.

Pour into lolly moulds and pop into the freezer until frozen. Take out and enjoy as a healthy evening or hot summer's day treat!

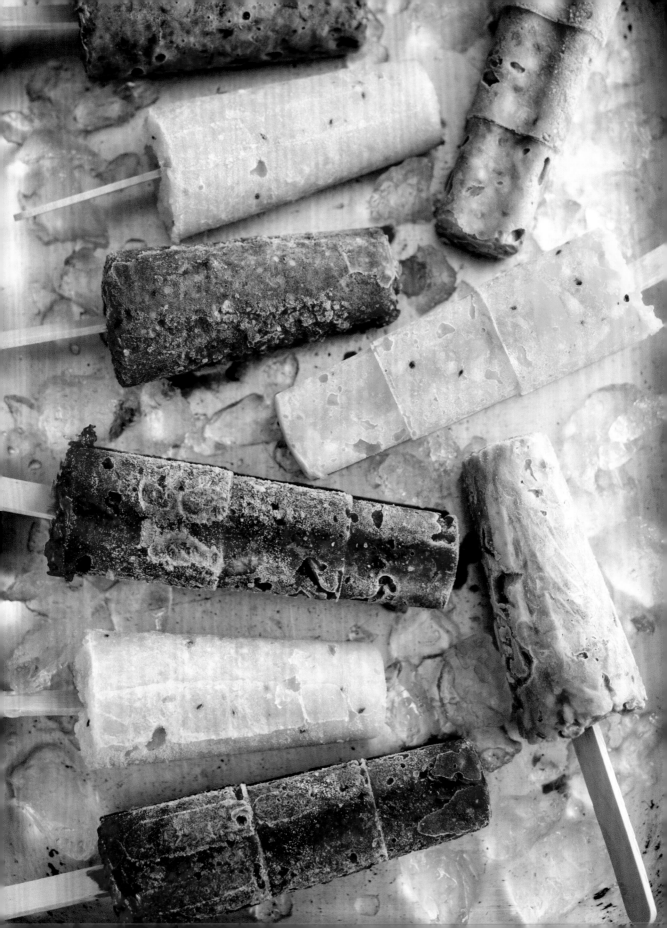

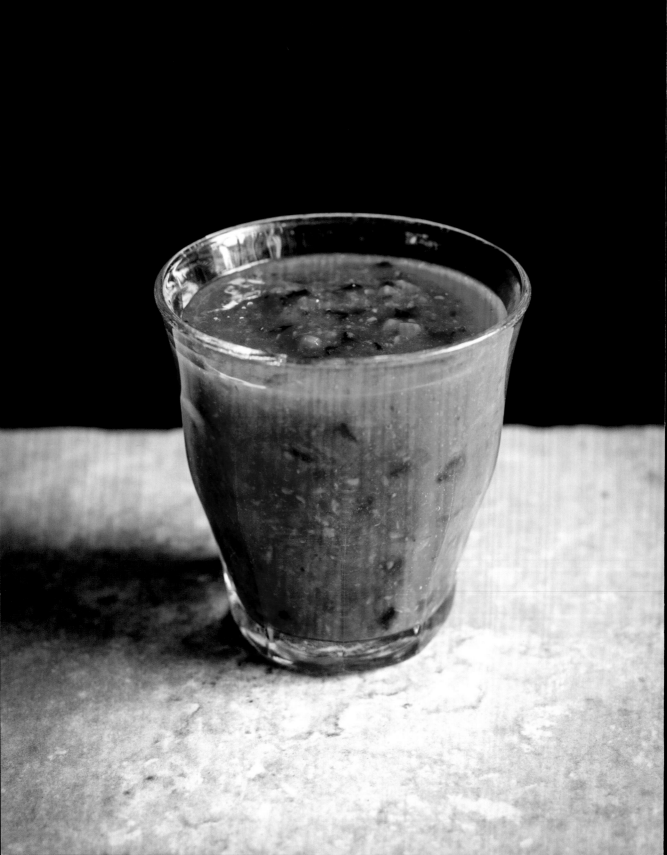

SMOOTHIES

The world of Viking mythology is filled with incredibly rich sagas of the Norse gods, witches and Valkyries. The centre of the Viking Cosmos is the giant tree Yggdrasil, which holds up the nine worlds, the home of gods, humans and all spiritual beings. For the Vikings, the sagas, the gods and their beliefs were not about finding salvation from this world but instead were about bringing to them power, strength, resilience and wisdom to rule themselves. Each Viking deity has qualities that will serve you greatly. Each smoothie incorporates specific qualities and is named after the Norse god that embodies those qualities.

A veg- and fruit-packed smoothie makes a great afternoon snack, whether it's a training or a rest day. They're also very good for breakfast, particularly if you're not much of a breakfast person, though I'd recommend supplementing them with a handful of nuts, or a boiled egg, to provide additional protein and fat to keep you energized and feeling full until lunch.

I blend all my smoothies with cold still water, to get them to that drinkable smooth consistency, without any lumps. It's all in the name. Chop, blitz and drink!

Always use whole fruits, never juice. If you use juice, you are mostly just getting the fruit sugar, and losing out on the fibre and vitamins and minerals that come from the actual fruit itself.

All the smoothie recipes serve one person, unless otherwise stated.

LOKI'S BERRY MADNESS: TO KEEP FIGHTING FIT

Loki is the trickster god, an extremely clever and immensely powerful magician, and the most dangerous deity in Norse mythology. All the ingredients in this smoothie are packed with antioxidants, which help to stop cell damage caused by oxidants, free radicals in the environment, food, everywhere – which is why it is so important to have a diet high in antioxidants.

70G BLUEBERRIES

70G RASPBERRIES

5 STRAWBERRIES, HALVED, TOPS CUT OFF

70G MANGO

A THUMB-SIZE PIECE OF GINGER, PEELED AND ROUGHLY CHOPPED

Put all the ingredients into your blender, add a splash of water and whizz to a pulp, adding more water as necessary to get the right smoothie consistency.

Pour into a glass and drink up, Viking!

FREYA'S FRUITY FIGHTER: FOR ENERGY & POWER

Freya is the goddess of war and death as well as the goddess of love, fertility, beauty and lust. She is wild, untamed and seeks to obtain what she desires no matter what. She is powerful and loving. Spinach is loaded with tons and tons of nutrients, providing protein, iron, vitamins and minerals. The benefits of spinach are so vast that you should have a lot of it in your diet. One of its benefits is that spinach helps to build up muscles by speeding the body's conversion of protein into muscle mass, making you strong and powerful!

1 PLUM

½ AN ORANGE

A HANDFUL OF SPINACH, WASHED

10 ALMONDS, SKIN ON, CHOPPED

4 STRAWBERRIES, HALVED, TOPS CUT OFF

70G BLUEBERRIES

Put all the ingredients into your blender, add a splash of water and whizz to a pulp, adding more water as necessary to get the right smoothie consistency.

Pour into a glass and drink up, Viking!

THOR'S THUNDER: FOR NERVES & MUSCLES

Thor is the god of thunder and the indefatigable defender of the gods and their fortress. His courage and sense of duty are unshakeable and his physical strength is virtually unmatched. Beetroot is absolutely packed with amazingness! Fibre, folate, manganese, vitamin C and iron. When you combine these nutrients, the benefits are greatly improved blood flow to your muscles, improving your muscle endurance and athletic performance.

½ A MEDIUM COOKED BEETROOT

A HANDFUL OF SPINACH, WASHED

½ AN ORANGE

1 SMALL BANANA, CHOPPED

Put all the ingredients into your blender, add a splash of water and whizz to a pulp, adding more water as necessary to get the right smoothie consistency.

Pour into a glass and drink up, Viking!

ODIN'S GREEN & MEAN: FOR BRAIN & BODY

Odin is the chief deity in Norse mythology. He is the god of life and death, poetry and wisdom. Each night his two ravens, Huginn (Thought) and Muninn (Memory), whisper all the world's news into his ears. Spirulina is a natural blue-green algae and a proper Viking power food. Almost 70% of its dry weight consists of complete protein, and the rest consists mostly of essential fatty acids. It's high in vitamins and minerals like calcium, iodine and zinc, and studies suggest that it is amazing for your brain. It improves cognitive performance, keeps your brain sharp, resists ageing, and protects it from the brain cells' death, damage and from degenerative diseases.

100G SPINACH, WASHED

3 BROCCOLI STEMS, ROUGHLY CHOPPED

70G BLUEBERRIES

½ AN AVOCADO

1 TBSP FLAXSEEDS

1 TSP SPIRULINA POWDER

Put all the ingredients into your blender, add a splash of water and whizz to a pulp, adding more water as necessary to get the right smoothie consistency.

Pour into a glass and drink up, Viking!

IDUN'S GOLDEN GOODNESS: FOR SKIN & ENERGY

Idun is the goddess of youth. She was the guardian of the golden apples; apples that kept the Gods immortal. Pineapple contains bromelain, which is anti-inflammatory and anti-swelling, and can aid in keeping your skin soft and smooth. Carrots are high in beta-carotene, an antioxidant that protects the skin and repairs skin tissue.

A 1CM THICK SLICE OF FRESH PINEAPPLE

1 ROYAL GALA APPLE, CORED AND CHOPPED (KEEP THE SKIN ON, IT'S EXTREMELY NUTRITIOUS)

½ TSP GROUND TURMERIC

½ MEDIUM CARROT, CHOPPED

70G BLUEBERRIES

Put all the ingredients into your blender, add a splash of water and whizz to a pulp, adding more water as necessary to get the right smoothie consistency.

Pour into a glass and drink up, Viking!

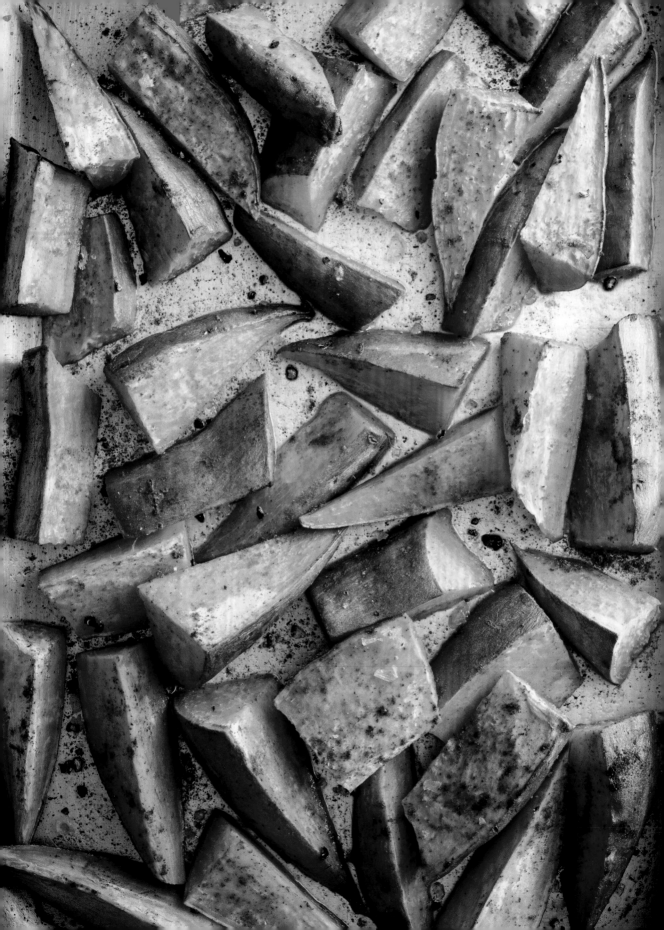

SOMETIMES CARBS

Here are some great options for your Post-training Meals: you can add these to any of the Anytime recipes to pack them full of enough energy to boost you after a workout.

This list may seem simple, but referring back to it makes it easier to keep your post-training recipes interesting by mixing things up and swapping one Sometimes Carb for another. This way you won't get bored!

Feel free to play around with flavours and textures. Fried onion, garlic and ginger are fantastic added to any of these Sometimes Carbs, as are spices like paprika, curry powder, ground cinnamon, cayenne and dried chillies. Fresh chopped herbs like coriander, parsley, dill, basil and chives can also be stirred through to boost the flavour.

Legumes (by which I mean beans, peas, lentils) are Sometimes Carbs, therefore you would normally have them as part of your Post-training Meals. However, legumes are also a really good source of protein (as well as being high in fibre, vitamins and minerals), which makes them a great choice for vegetarians. Therefore, if you are a vegetarian, you should consider these a protein.

Healthy eating is not complicated. It's more that we can lack inspiration or motivation to constantly come up with new things to eat. I understand that completely, and I hope that I am helping to remove any tedium from the process and make choosing a balanced nutritious meal easier.

We are in this together. Clanship all the way!

SWEET POTATOES – FOUR WAYS

I love sweet potatoes: they are high in fibre, the antioxidant beta-carotene, and a whole host of vitamins and minerals. They are naturally sweet and, unlike regular potatoes, they count as one of your five a day. What's not to love! With these four methods below, there's no excuse for not eating them.

Average portion = 1 medium sweet potato

MASH

Peel the sweet potato and cut into small chunks. Put into a pan with enough water to cover, and a pinch of salt if you like. Simmer until soft (stick a knife in to check if you're not sure – when it slides through, it's ready). Remove from the heat and mash immediately, adding butter and a splash of goat's milk if you like, and seasoning with salt, pepper, and any other spices such as nutmeg or cinnamon. It won't be completely smooth but should have a good creamy texture. Taste and add more seasoning if you want.

CHARGRILLED

Peel a medium sweet potato and cut into 1cm rounds. Grill in a hot pan with a teaspoon of oil for 10 minutes, or until soft and caramelized. Season with salt and pepper.

FRIES

Preheat the oven to 200°C/180°C fan/gas 6. Peel the sweet potato or scrub with a vegetable brush, and cut lengthways into long thin wedges, like fries. They don't have to be perfect – the more wonkily they're cut, the better they'll taste. Line a roasting tray with foil. Put the fries in the tray and drizzle over some rapeseed oil, then season with salt and pepper and any other seasoning you like (paprika is good). Mix together with your hands, making sure the potatoes get nicely coated, and roast for 30–40 minutes, turning if necessary, until they are crisp and caramelized at the edges and soft and juicy within.

BAKED

Preheat the oven to 200°C/180°C fan/gas 6. Peel the sweet potato or scrub with a vegetable brush. Line a roasting tray with foil. If you like, you can rub the potato with a little rapeseed oil and sprinkle it with salt. Bake in the hot oven for around 45 minutes to an hour – the time will depend on the size of your potato. Remove and slice into your potato, mashing and seasoning its flesh with salt and pepper. Delicious with a dollop of goat's yoghurt with some horseradish mixed into it.

QUINOA

Although it's cooked like a grain, quinoa is actually a seed. If you want to add extra flavour to your quinoa, use 240ml of vegetable or chicken stock instead of water when cooking it.

90G QUINOA

240ML WATER

A PINCH OF SEA SALT

Rinse the quinoa and put into a pan with the water and a pinch of salt.

Bring to the boil, then reduce the heat and let simmer for 15–20 minutes.

GREAT WITH: Roasted Vegetables with Feta & Seeds (see page 167), Seared Seabass with Spicy Red Pepper Salsa (see page 162).

BROWN RICE

A wholegrain, unprocessed brown rice is nuttier than white rice, more filling, and requires a longer cooking time.

100G BROWN RICE

500ML WATER

A PINCH OF SEA SALT

Put the rice into a pan with the water and a pinch of salt.

Bring to the boil, then reduce the heat and let simmer for 35 minutes.

Turn off the heat and let the rice sit in the pan with the lid on for 10 minutes. This helps it absorb the last of the liquid that is in the pan, making it light and fluffy when you serve it.

GREAT WITH: Salsa Chicken (see page 168), Thor-red Salmon (see page 173).

HULLED BARLEY

Barley is an amazing wholegrain and has always been popular in the Nordic countries. It's very high in fibre, vitamins, mineral, and antioxidants. So mix it up, and try hulled barley instead of rice.

100G BARLEY

500ML WATER

Soak the barley overnight in water.

Drain and rinse the barley, then put into a pan with the 500ml of water.

Bring to the boil, then reduce the heat and simmer for 45 minutes, until tender.

GREAT WITH: Seared Seabass with Spicy Red Pepper Salsa (see page 162), Cajun Goat's Milk Yoghurt Chicken (page 170).

RICE NOODLES

These can range from thin vermicelli noodles, to thicker round noodles and flat ribbons. Always read the packet instructions, as the cooking methods may vary: the steps below are for dried vermicelli.

50G RICE NOODLES

500ML BOILING WATER

Place the rice noodles in a medium heatproof bowl and pour the boiling water over them. Cover with a clean tea towel or a plate to stop the steam escaping.

Stir the noodles every couple of minutes to loosen them up.

When the strands have separated and the noodles are soft, they are ready (around 4–5 minutes). Drain thoroughly.

GREAT WITH: Tangy Stir-fried Tofu & Vegetables (see page 160).

BLACK TURTLE BEANS

These beans are so versatile and they're also high in fibre, antioxidants, vitamins and minerals. They are a great source of protein for vegetarians! You can add aromatics such as half an onion, a bashed garlic clove, a stick of celery, a bay leaf, or a dried chilli to the water when cooking, for added flavour.

100G DRIED BLACK TURTLE BEANS

500ML WATER

Soak the turtle beans overnight (or for at least 8 hours).

Drain the beans and rinse in fresh water.

Put into a pan with the 500ml of water. Bring to the boil, then reduce the heat and simmer for an hour, until tender.

GREAT WITH: Cajun-spiced Chicken with Halloumi (see page 163).

GREEN & BROWN LENTILS

A wonderful source of carbohydrate and protein, great for vegetarians, lentils also contain calcium, phosphorus, iron and B vitamins – and they count towards your five a day! Green and brown lentils retain their shape, but tend to take longer to cook than other varieties – though they can be pre-soaked to reduce the cooking time. As with the black beans (see left), you can add extra aromatics to the water for additional flavour.

100G DRIED GREEN OR BROWN LENTILS

400ML WATER

Rinse the lentils, then drain and place in a pan with the water.

Bring to the boil, then reduce the heat and simmer for around 30 minutes, until the lentils are tender.

GREAT WITH: Roasted Tuna Steak and Mixed Vegetables (see page 164), Chicken & Golden Cauliflower Rice (see page 166).

» KNOW THY LABEL

Always read the nutritional table on the back of food packets!

Less than 5g of sugars per 100g is low in sugar, which is what you should aim for.

The higher fibre content the better: food high in fibre has more than 5g per 100g.

High salt is 1.5g of salt per 100g; low is less than 0.3 per 100g.

Also check the ingredients. These are listed in order from the highest amount to the lowest, with any allergens highlighted in bold. Check that what you are buying is actually what you are buying i.e. the first ingredient in a chickpea burger should be chickpeas (often the first ingredient is potatoes; cheap and bulky and then the chickpea comes later: not good). Always know what you are buying.

WEEKLY VIKING TRAINING AND NUTRITION PLAN AND PROGRESS TRACKER

Opposite is an example of a weekly plan for your nutrition and training. The most important thing to remember is that Vikings are always prepared.

When you train affects what you should eat. For example, whether you train in the afternoon or the evening will inform what you should eat for lunch.

Points to remember:

>> On Training and Madness days you should have Sometimes Carbs (see pages 224–9) in the morning as well as **after you train.**

>> If you train before breakfast, you should have a Training Day Breakfast (see pages 106–15) **after you train** plus Sometimes Carbs for lunch to fully replenish your energy stores. (See Lunch and Dinner, Training Days, pages 118–57.)

>> The rest of the time, use recipes from any of the Anytime Meals, Snacks and Salads (see pages 158, 204, 216). There's lots of goodness to choose from!

>> The whole point of the Viking Method is that it shouldn't feel like you're compromising or making concessions – the opposite, in fact. The recipes in the book are delicious, filling and varied, with lots of options, and they taste as good as they are good for you. So 'cheating' doesn't need to come into it. If you want to have a slice of pizza or a piece of cake, you can make that decision without being told you're allowed to because it's your 'cheat day'. Take responsibility for your actions. Empower yourself. Be a Viking.

After the first week, check on your previous time before you do the Madness again. And every week, work to smash that time.

When you do the Before Challenge, just do it. It doesn't matter how many reps you get. Do not negatively analyse it or judge yourself.

THE VIKING CHALLENGE	REPS
Before Date:	
After Date:	

THE VIKING MADNESS	TIME
Week 1	
Week 2	
Week 3	
Week 4	

Sample Meal Plan	Monday If you train before lunch	Tuesday If you train before dinner	Weds Rest day	Thursday If you train before breakfast	Friday If you train before lunch	Saturday If you train before dinner	Sunday Rest day
Morning	**Breakfast** Immune Injection Porridge **Training** Programme 1	**Breakfast** Iron Energy Boom Porridge	**Breakfast** Take Off! Omelette **Snacks** Apple with cinnamon	**Training** Programme 1 **Breakfast** Chia Porridge with Blueberries & Cinnamon	**Breakfast** Antioxidant Shot Porridge **Training** Programme 2	**Breakfast** Chia Porridge with Blueberries & Cinnamon	**Breakfast** Veggie Frittatas & Greens
Midday	**Lunch** Pesto Chicken & Sweet Potato One-tray Wonder **Snacks** Idunn's Golden Goodness Smoothie	**Lunch** Chicken Fajita Salad **Snacks** 1 Viking Baller Ball **Training** Programme 2	**My Ugly Lunch box** Salmon & Super Greens **Snacks** Celery & cucumber with hummus	**Lunch** All-day Breakfast Wrap **Snacks** Freya's Fruity Fighter Smoothie	**Lunch** Chicken with Curried Scrambled Eggs, Lentils & Good Stuff **Snacks** Apple with cinnamon	**Lunch** Sirloin Steak with Filled Portobello Mushrooms **Snacks** Loki's Berry Madness **Training** Viking Madness	**Lunch** Roasted Tuna Steak & Mixed Vegetables **Snacks** Odin's Green & Mean Smoothie
Evening	**Dinner** Seared Seabass with Spicy Red Pepper Salsa	**Dinner** Icelandic Lamb Stew	**Dinner** Chicken Stir-fry with Edamame	**Dinner** Chicken & Golden Cauliflower Rice	**Dinner** Icelandic-Inspired Poached Cod	**Dinner** Cajun Goat's Milk Yoghurt Chicken, The Warrior Pasta Salad	**Dinner** Chicken Skewers with Satay Sauce

Meal Plan	Monday If you train before lunch	Tueday If you train before dinner	Weds Rest day	Thursday If you train before breakfast	Friday If you train before lunch	Saturday If you train before dinner	Sunday Rest day
Morning	Breakfast Training Programme 1	Breakfast	Breakfast Snacks	Training Programme 1 Breakfast	Breakfast Training Programme 2	Breakfast	Breakfast
Midday	Lunch Snacks	Lunch Snacks Training Programme 2	My Ugly Lunch box Snacks	Lunch Snacks	Lunch Snacks	Lunch Snacks Training Viking Madness	Lunch Snacks
Evening	Dinner	Dinner	Dinner	Dinner	Dinner	Dinner	Dinner

VIKING MENTAL POINTER

YOU ARE NOT GOING TO TAKE LESS
WHEN YOU KNOW YOU DESERVE MORE.
YOU ARE NOT GOING TO SAY YES WHEN
YOUR GUT IS TELLING YOU THAT
YOU SHOULD SAY NO.
YOU ARE NOT GOING TO DEMONSTRATE
TO PEOPLE THAT THEIR TIME IS MORE
VALUABLE THAN YOUR TIME.
WHAT YOU ARE GOING TO DO IS STAND
UP FOR YOURSELF. BE DEMANDING.
TURN YOUR VOLUME UP. TAKE UP SPACE.
HAVE SOME STAMINA.
YOU ARE GOING TO DO WHAT YOU
SAID YOU WOULD DO.
YOU WILL NOT GIVE UP.
YOU'VE GOT THIS.

INDEX

RECIPE INDEX

ACKNOWLEDGEMENTS

We all create our own future, some of us consciously and others unconsciously. When it is done consciously, the future is never a surprise.

It is like baking. You get the recipe for a banana bread, you buy all the ingredients, you do the steps, you put it into the oven and out comes, of course, a banana bread. If you are living unconsciously you do all of that, then take out the banana bread and you are absolutely baffled as to why it isn't a chocolate cake. It is a complete surprise.

You have to understand that if you want a chocolate cake you have to get the recipe, the ingredients, the steps, for a chocolate cake! That is how life works.

If you want a certain future, then you have to consciously create that future. You have to plan for that future, take action for that future.

I am so incredibly thankful, I feel so fortunate, and my heart is so filled with gratitude. If someone were to ask me, 'How are you?' I would say, 'I'm blessed.'

But I am not surprised. I am not going: 'How the hell did this happen? How am I an author?' This book is a goal come true.

This book was a conscious creation, a goal set when I started the Viking Method. To write a book that would give all of you tools for long-term growth, wellness, strength, success, contentment and self-love, both physically and mentally.

But I couldn't have written this book without the support, commitment, vision and expertise of these amazing people:

My agency, the Blair Partnership, Neil, Zoe and my wonderful agent Amy.

My incredible publisher, Emily, and the team at Penguin Life, Natalie and Josie.

My dearest Emma and Alex for making the book look so slayingly beautiful.

My superwomen; Nicole and Amanda.

Philip, Tim, Sam and Edward for shooting the most badass photos of me, and Keti and Veronika for making me look so badass in them.

The amazing twosome, Sophie and Annie, for editing the book with me, making it perfect.

Jacqui and Vicki-Marie for spreading the Viking message with me when I was starting out and for being such awesome friends.

Why Projects, Nick, Stephen and Jon for bringing forth the language and the style of the Viking Method.

Sonia, Ashley, Susanne, Dayen, my ultimate Vikings, who have been with me from the word go and have never left my side.

Laura Bradbury for your expertise and wonderful creations.

Sveta, my beautiful angel and my wonderful Lilja Birna, for bringing the Viking Method with me all over the world.

My mother, Birna. For helping me, guiding me, inspiring me, making this book a reality with me.

My Raven. You can always stay. Actually, please always stay.

My family and my friends. I love you.

To my Viking Clan, both near and far, in person, online, on social media, I namaslay you. The slay in me always sees the slay in you. I truly have the Best Clan.

And finally, to all of you that have bought this book, I thank you.

And welcome you.

It's so wonderful to have you with us.

You are a Viking now.

Know your life. Know your future.

Yours in Berserkness always,
Svava.